WHERE YOUR MIND GOES, YOU GO

REVISED, VOLUME 1

"As an owner of a network marketing company, I've read and referred my share of 'self-help' books to hundreds of people throughout the years; so I'm a believer in the process and also understand how hard it can be to take in what many authors suggest. Sometimes, it's too much. This is exactly why I love Where Your Mind Goes, You Go; it's a very simple, day-by-day, practical application. Clark has you read one day at a time and also makes you 'take action' and do something. I highly suggest reading both volumes one and two and then reread them…the material is that good and easily digestible for anyone, honestly."

Jack Fallon
CEO, Total Life Changes

"As a bestselling author and fitness professional myself, I understand the value of working to constantly improve by finding resources to helping the process. Clark's dedication to helping people, myself included, and the fact he has that coaching in print, is a testament to the fact that he is committed to helping others achieve their best in life. Both volumes of Where Your Mind Goes, You Go are a great resource for anyone inter-ested in personal and physical development. It's a MUST HAVE in your self-help library."

John Rowley Author
Old School New Body

Clark and I have been friends since childhood. I've watched him achieve in everything he does in spite of being told by others that he couldn't. I have also watched him refine his knowledge and behaviors that lead to success to the point where I believe Clark can do anything he puts his mind to. It was very exciting for me to see his book for the first time because it captures the essence of the attitude and behaviors that I have watched him practice for years in a clear and easy to understand format. Anyone who puts the information in this book into practice cannot fail.

Richard G. King
Technology Solutions Manager
Major US Corporation

Clark Bartram - "America's Most Trusted Fitness Professional" - is an ISSA Master Trainer who has helped thousands of men and women transform their bodies and their lives. As co-host of ESPN's Kiana's Flex Appeal, and his own fitness television show, American Health & Fitness, he has inspired millions.

As an actor, Clark has played the iconic super-hero Batman in the cult classic Batman: Dead End and the leading role as Orin Jericho in the feature film Hunter Prey. He has appeared on the cover 9of over 130 fitness publications making him one of the most successful fitness models in the industry and he is a regular contributor to numerous fitness magazines. Clark has appeared on Home Shopping Network and QVC selling home fitness products branded with his name. Beside his bestseller, Where Your Mind Goes, You Go, Clark has authored the how-to guide You Too Can Be a Fitness Model and Spiritually Fit, a Fitness Program You Can Have Faith In.

Clark was actively involved with Prison Fellowship's Operation Starting Line and has worked with the Bill Graham Evangelistic Association as an emcee for the Franklin Graham Crusades. He continues to travel the country speaking at various events motivation people to "think about what they think about."
In addition to his full-time career and public speaking, Clark is a devoted husband and father.

For more information
about Clark Bartram, visit his Web site at
www.clarkbartram.com

WHERE YOUR MIND GOES, YOU GO

A MENTAL JOURNEY TOWARD A HEALTHY BODY AND A SUCCESSFUL LIFE, REVISED, VOLUME 1

BY CLARK BARTRAM

INDIGORIVER
PUBLISHING

Where Your Mind Goes, You Go: A Mental Journey Toward a Healthy Body and a Successful Life

Photo Credits: Clark Bartram and Taylor Bartram Photography, *www.taylorbartramphotography.com*

Editors: Kathryn Middleton

Cover Design: Jason Kauffmann / Firelight Interactive / firelightinteractive.com

Indigo River Publishing
3 West Garden Street Ste. 352
Pensacola, FL 32502
www.indigoriverpublishing.com

Ordering Information:
Quantity sales: Special discounts are available on quantity purchases by corporations, associations, and others. For details, contact the publisher at the address above.

Orders by U.S. trade bookstores and wholesalers: Please contact the publisher at the address above.

Printed in the United States of America

Library of Congress Control Number: 2015954261

ISBN: 9780996233033)

First Edition

With Indigo River Publishing, you can always expect great books, strong voices, and meaningful messages. Most importantly, you'll always find … words worth reading.

INTRODUCTION

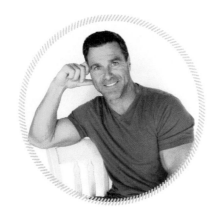

. . . your thoughts and words are directly responsible for the successes and failures in your life.

WITH MORE THAN TWO DECADES of experience in the health and fitness industry, I've learned a few things about losing fat, sculpting abs, and eating right for optimum health. For years, I've work directly with clients and helped men and women transform their bodies—and their lives. After working with literally thousands of everyday people, I am not looking to pad my resume with names. Instead, I am attempting to connect with people who understand (or want to understand) the bigger picture.

The thing is we get it wrong in America. Our barometer has always been the scale, the mirror, and how our clothes fit. Yes, I understand why, but I KNOW we have it backwards. I wish the barometer was gauged from the inside—things like cellular health, bone density, heart and lung function, all of the reports you get from the doctor, as well as emotional and mental health. I agree a good-looking, mus-

Scales cannot measure what an amazing person you are...

cular, toned body is a great byproduct of exercise but should never be the end all, be all. If we let the scale become what gives us joy, we are in for an up-and-down rollercoaster ride. Scales are seldom accurate. Scales cannot measure what an amazing person you are, what a great parent, spouse, friend, employee, or boss you are. It can only tell you a number that means nothing at the end of the day.

Many of you may be surprised by why I wrote this book. It wasn't because I was some psychology major in college. I didn't even go to college. It wasn't because I felt like I had information that people needed to hear since when I first wrote this, I felt very inadequate and didn't think I had anything of any importance to say. No, this book was born out of one of the darkest and scariest times of my life.

I had a contract with a company that licensed my name and image for products that were going to be sold on HSN, and I had made several trips to Tampa to sell these products live on HSN. I am a very confident guy. I knew the products I had worked. I knew the price was right. I wasn't nervous going on live TV on a channel that reaches upwards of ninety-five million homes. But then something happened.

I was standing off the side of the stage as the host was giving me a rather impressive introduction. My earpiece was in. I could hear the line producers calling camera shots and talking about different technical things when suddenly my whole entire body began to tingle from head to toe. My tongue felt like it was swelling up, and my palms were so sweaty there were almost puddles forming on the floor. The announcer was building to a crescendo, and I thought to myself, "*I have to get out of here. There is no way I can go out there.*" And I almost ran out of the backstage entrance, but when she said my name, I just went out there and battled through the discomfort I felt.

The show actually went well. I didn't sell out of product, but I did well enough that I was invited back for another show with another product. A few months passed, and I went back as an old pro. I did several airings, and eventually the sign that every product pitch person works for appeared on the screen: Sold Out! Clark Bartram's 3D Ab was a hit, and big things were on the horizon. That night, I went to dinner, and directly across from me sat Frankie Avalon, who also had just come from HSN where he was selling a joint pain formula. I had finally made it to the pinnacle. I was there. The stars were aligned for me to shoot to the stratosphere, and I was going to help a lot of people and make a lot of money.

I was flying home excited because my next airing was already booked. I was watching *Million Dollar Baby* and didn't have a care in the world. Then suddenly, I thought to myself, "*I feel like I'm going to die.*" My heart was beating out of control. I was hyperventilating, my feet and tongue felt as if they were swelling again, and my palms were sweating even worse than the last time.

I was thinking to myself, "*Oh my God. I'm having a heart attack. I need some oxygen!*" But I did nothing but sit there paralyzed by fear. I had no idea what to do. My next thought was, "*I'm going to jump*

The stars were aligned for me to shoot to the stratosphere...

out of the airplane!" That's not even an exaggeration. I was honestly thinking of jumping because I wanted out of there so badly, and we weren't landing in Dallas for another hour and a half. As I tried to breathe, I began to pray. I searched for music to calm me down. I wanted to find someone right then to talk to that could explain to me what was happening, but I was frozen in fear.

Finally, after the plane touched down in Dallas, I called my wife as I sat on the floor outside the train that takes you from one terminal to the next. I told her there was no way I was getting on another plane. I just couldn't imagine going through that again. However, I needed to get home. I couldn't drive, and deep down I didn't want this unknown fear to control me. My wife patiently talked to me until the doors closed on the plane, and I finally made it home. That night, I had a conference call I hosted, and as they were introducing me, the fear jumped all over me again. I could barely make it through the call. My voice was shaky, and I didn't perform to the best of my ability.

I was scheduled to go back to HSN for another airing of 3D Abs. They were excited about me and my potential. Problem was, I couldn't do it. I was fearful of freaking out again, so I asked my manager if they could get someone to go in my place. I told him in confidence that I was having some emotional issues I needed to sort out, and I begged that he keep it private. I told him that eventually I would be good to go. A replacement went to sell in my absence and didn't do well. The product hardly sold at all. HSN immediately pulled my deal, and my company

I just couldn't imagine going through that again...

let me go. My secret didn't remain between my manager and me. The whole company knew that "Clark was crazy," and that was the end of what could have been a very lucrative deal in my career.

I was lost. I had no clue what to do, so I made an appointment with a counselor. I remember walking into the building where his office was, and the hallway seemed like it was a mile long. I could barely bring myself to walk down there to face whatever it was that had me losing the very thing that I had counted on my whole life: my confidence.

Now I was too scared to walk down a hallway...

My confidence got me everything I ever accomplished in life. It was what makes me a great dad, an awesome coach, and a great personal trainer. It made me think I could write a book, and I had. My confidence was the reason I rose to the top of a very cluttered industry of models who all wanted to land the next cover or get the next endorsement contract. I consistently got jobs for over twenty years because I was confident. Now I was too scared to walk down a hallway to hear a man tell me I may not be as awesome as I always believed I was.

I had long and amazing sessions with Charlie, an older gentleman who was an athlete. The first day, he showed up in jeans and flip-flops, and we talked about "guy stuff." Throughout our sessions, we talked about my childhood. We discussed the fact that my kids were growing up. He taught me about the lifecycle phases that we all go through at different stages of our lives. Eventually, Charlie helped me understand I was fine.

Where the mind goes, the
man follows...

I was going to be okay, but there were going to be some deep issues I was going to have to work through. This took time.

Through this, my quest for knowledge became fierce. I knew I had some areas in my life that I could clean up. I knew I was engaging in conversations and activities that were not conducive to being a totally healthy person. I realized my thoughts and feelings contributed to my successes and failures. So I educated myself, and that is exactly what I needed. I saw Charlie a couple times a week. I read every book I could get my hands on. I watched some great ministry on TV. I sat in the front row at church every week, Wednesday included. I searched for answers everywhere I could. I didn't want to just take pills. I knew that I needed to give some good old positive thinking a chance first. So I grew.

Then something else happened. I was innocently watching Joyce Meyer on television when she said, "Where the mind goes, the man follows." Something in my spirit jumped and said, "*That's the title to your book!*" Then I thought to myself, "*What book? I'm not writing a book.*"

After a moment, I said out loud, "Okay, I guess I'm going to write a book." I got up off the couch and started to write right then. I didn't wait. I didn't think about it. I started writing immediately, and I didn't stop for two weeks. I rarely left the house. I was skipping workouts. I felt like this book was happening to me. I wasn't writing it. It was literally happening to me. The knowledge was pouring into my soul, and it came out my fingers and onto the computer.

This book needed to come out of me. It was meant to happen. I don't care that I lost my HSN deal and contract with my company because I wrote a book that is changing thousands of lives around the world. So the most important lesson I can teach you from experience is this: Nothing will ever work for you until you understand that your thoughts and words are directly responsible for your successes and failures. The mind is powerful and is an amazing tool when it comes to your fitness goals. In fact, you cannot live a healthy life while focusing only on the body. Fitness only comes from working on the mind, body, *and* spirit. Having a free mind frees the body to engage in activity that will manifest in a healthy and vibrant existence. A free mind opens the spirit, opens the heart, and opens every possibility to experience TOTAL health.

With that in mind, I put together a simple, yet very effective thirty-day mental journey to help you take control and move yourself in a positive direction toward whatever goals you have. If you use this program every day for the next thirty days, it will absolutely have a significant impact, as these concepts have had with me. There's nothing in this book that I haven't done for myself over the years and I believe it will give you the tools to make your life better. Trust me.

Your mind is a powerful tool you can use to change your life. So do yourself a favor and fully engage in this process. Great things are going to happen to you.

Fitness only comes from working on the mind, body, and spirit.

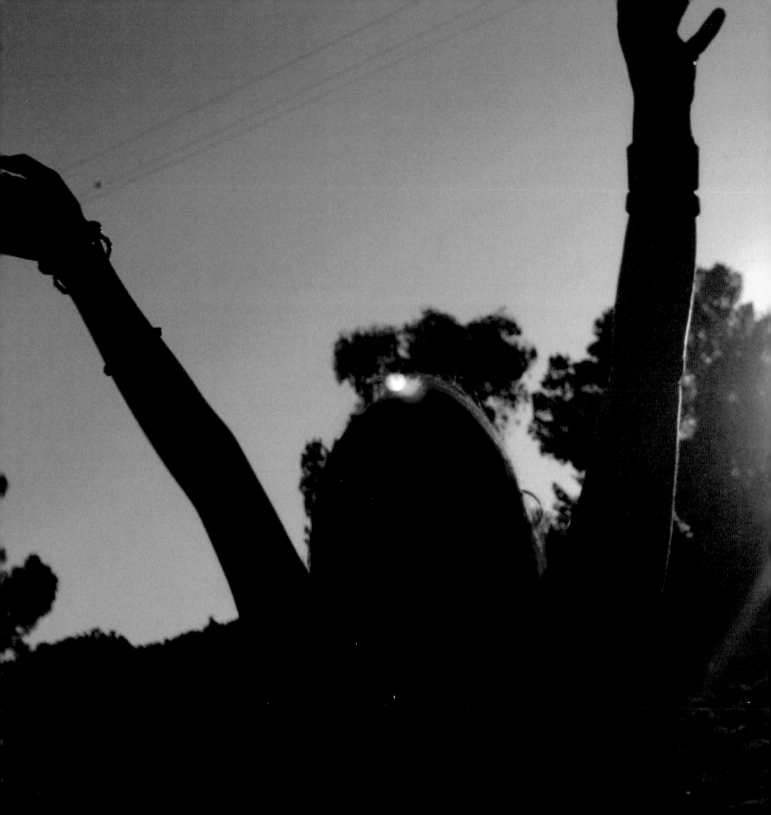

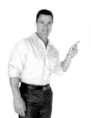

IMPORTANT

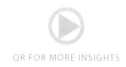

HOW TO READ THIS BOOK!

QR FOR MORE INSIGHTS

I **KNOW YOU'LL BE TEMPTED** to finish this book in a single day, but don't! This isn't a thriller or a mystery where you have to find out what happens next. It doesn't even have a beginning, middle, or end. This is unlike any other book you'll ever read. It's a carefully thought-out, step-by-step guidebook to the incredibly exciting story of your life, as lived each day for thirty days in a row.

You don't want to overload your mind with too much information, so it's important that you read no more than one lesson per day for the next thirty days. Take the time to allow each new lesson to sink into your conscious and subconscious minds so you can incorporate it into your ongoing process of personal growth. You owe it to yourself to do this right!

Here's all you have to do: When you get up in the morning, read the information for that particular day. Spend a few minutes with it

. . . read no more than one lesson per day for the next thirty days.

and consider the questions in the "Think about this!" section. Then, throughout the day, follow the directions for putting the day's lesson into practice. If it's a simple affirmation, for example, say it out loud as often as you can. At some point, take some time out and answer the "Think about this!" questions in writing. Set aside at least thirty minutes for this. I promise, you'll be glad you did! And finally, at the end of each day before you go to sleep, read the information again along with your answers and reflect on how it's helping you become a better person.

In each chapter, there will be two QR codes. The first will lead you to a video in which I discuss each day's lesson further and give you extra knowledge and information. Admittedly, sometimes I find writing hard, but speaking comes very easily to me, especially when I want to get a point across with information as sensitive as what we are dealing with in this book. So, I recommend you take advantage of these videos, as they will certainly give you more to think about.

The second QR code will take you to a related exercise for that day. If you are looking to improve your fitness along with your mind, as you should be doing, then these will help you with that goal. Each exercise connects to that day's lesson and will be easy enough that anyone can do it. If you are a beginner, you can just focus on the exercises I give you. If you are further along with your fitness, you can always add the exercise to your workout, taking my advice in account with your current regimen.

If you are unfamiliar with QR codes, it is just a code you can scan to be sent to a video or a link. You can simply download a QR code reader in any app store. Hold your phone over the code on the lesson and up pops the video or exercise. What we've effectively done is bridge old- and new-school publishing with this technology. Don't be afraid of it. If you are not too tech savvy, just have a teenager help you, and you will be well on your way into the twenty-first century.

DON'T DRINK THE POISON

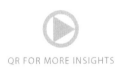

YOU MAY HAVE HEARD THE SAYING, "Refusing to forgive is like drinking poison and hoping it kills the other person." Forgiveness, believe it or not, could be the one thing standing in the way of the healthy, vibrant body you've been longing for or any other positive goal you may have. I realize that forgiveness is probably the hardest thing that any of us can do as human beings, but it's my opinion that, and this is the reason it's day one, forgiveness is the most powerful tool we have.

How do I define forgiveness? I can't. Sure, I can go grab a dictionary and give you a bunch of scholars' idea of what forgiveness is, but will that help? Probably not. So instead here's what I've learned about forgiveness in my own life: regardless of how you want to define it, forgiveness becomes freedom from a self-made prison in which we hold onto someone else's inability to treat us with the respect we

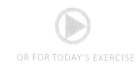

QR FOR TODAY'S EXERCISE

deserve or desire. We've all been hurt by people, either by what they said or what they did, but the thing we need to understand is that in most cases it was them that did it, not us, and we cannot control their actions. Hanging onto resentment will keep you captive to the memory of whatever it was that offended and hurt you so deeply. We cannot give people the freedom and privilege to continue to hurt us by not releasing them from our thoughts.

While I understand the feeling of wanting to wish ill will on an offender, I know for a fact that it only affects the person who's harboring the negative emotions. Hateful thoughts have to manifest themselves in some way, and they often manifest in the form of comfort eating, depression, and diseases.

Self-forgiveness, in my opinion, is the first place we need to start in forgiving others. We often times cannot forgive those who have hurt us because we blame ourselves for the experiences causing us pain, believing we asked for it or made it happen. You must understand that you never deserve to be hurt. People hurt others because they feel they need power, and these actions come from a person who is ignorant, less than realized, and doesn't have a fully developed thought process of compassion and love. It is never your fault, and until you forgive yourself for the blame you've placed on yourself, you will most likely be unable to forgive the transgressor—too caught up in your self-blame.

. . .forgiveness becomes freedom from a self-made prison. . .

Is the process of forgiving hard? Absolutely. Is it worth the effort? More than you can ever imagine. My recommendation is this: dig deep, be consistent, retrain your thoughts about that hurt, and use the pain to make yourself stronger. Encourage somebody else who may be experiencing the same painful process you have managed to live through and, when you make a positive impact, become thankful to your transgressors for bringing you so much power with the very acts they attempted to destroy you with. The ball has always been in your court and will remain there. It's up to you to pick it up, advance it down field, make forward progress, gain positive yards, and score a point or pass it off to someone who is there to help you along the way.

How about defining what forgiveness is to you? Write down your thoughts and feelings on how your pain can be something that is used to advance your life, not take it backward. Next, I want you to start trying to forgive everyone you are still harboring resentment toward. Exactly how you do all this is up to you. Who I am to tell you how to proceed? I'm working through my own stuff, if I'm being honest, and this book is part of that process. Each person must walk a different path and define his or her own process, but I believe it all begins with a true desire to heal, move forward, and accomplish mental freedom.

One thing you could do is reach out to these people and forgive them directly through a personal visit or phone call, but a card or an email would also suffice. If you can't even do that yet, you can also try to forgive them in your heart or start working through your pain through prayer, reading, and/or deep thought.

No matter what you choose, the bottom line is this: start TODAY with something that you feel will work for you and NEVER stop until you achieve the forgiveness and mental freedom you need to move forward at a consistent pace.

THINK ABOUT THIS!

What situations have caused you to resent others or feel bad about yourself? How long have you been harboring resentments? How can forgiving yourself and others help you free yourself to take more positive actions?

_____

_____

_____

_____

_____

_____

_____

_____

_____

_____

DAY **2**

LET OTHERS INSPIRE YOU

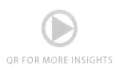

QR FOR MORE INSIGHTS

ILOVE QUOTES. THEY INSPIRE ME. They motivate me. They guide me. They show me that others have been in the same place and have somehow, against all odds, figured it out. Quotes can do the same for you. Here's a great quote for today to start you off. And I don't even know who said it!

> *"Whatever you hold in your mind will tend to occur in your life. If you continue to believe as you have always believed, you will continue to act as you have always acted. If you continue to act as you have always acted, you will continue to get what you have always gotten. If you want different results in your life or your work, all you have to do is change your mind."*
>
> —Anonymous

Today's message is short but powerful. Be sure to read the above quote over and over, aloud whenever possible, and think about how it applies to your life. Continue to do something like this daily. Find quotes that inspire you and then inspire others with those quotes. Tweet them, post them on social media, and just spread the words of people who have inspired you. Doing this causes a cascade of positivity and purging of negativity. People will either reciprocate or eliminate. By this, I mean that as people feel your outpouring of positivity, they may either encourage you or tell you to stop. Purge those negative people because you are evolving and they are stagnating, and we both know what happens in stagnant water … death.

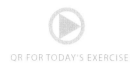

QR FOR TODAY'S EXERCISE

THINK ABOUT THIS!

What does the above quote mean to you? What other quotes inspire you to make great changes and get better results?

_____

_____

_____

_____

_____

_____

_____

_____

_____

_____

LIVE WITH A PURPOSE

EVERY SUCCESSFUL COMPANY HAS A mission statement to help keep it on track. Shouldn't successful people have the same thing?

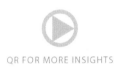

QR FOR MORE INSIGHTS

About fifteen years ago, I was challenged to create a personal statement of purpose. I didn't really get it until I actually wrote it out and saw the effect that it had on my life. Now, when I have a rough day, I repeat my mission statement in my head and ask myself, "Am I really living this? Do I mean it? Am I really this person?" Then, I can easily get out of my pity party, stop being negative, and enjoy the rewards of enriching someone else's life.

Your mission statement doesn't have to be long or complicated. My personal statement of purpose is "to positively and powerfully affect everyone I come into contact with." How did I come up with that? It took many days of deep thought, prayer, and consideration on who I am at the core. I don't expect you to get your statement on the first try, but I do want you to spend this day brainstorming ideas and working toward creating a concise statement that defines your mission to make a difference in life.

Keep working on it each day until you get a short statement that works for you and say it to yourself every day when you wake up. I guarantee that you'll never wake up on the wrong side of the bed again!

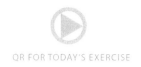

QR FOR TODAY'S EXERCISE

THINK ABOUT THIS!

Who are the people you admire the most? Can you write personal statements of purpose for your heroes? How can that help you write one for yourself?

_____
_____
_____
_____
_____
_____
_____
_____
_____
_____
_____

4

MAKE THE RIGHT MIND-SPIRIT-BODY CONNECTION

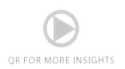

QR FOR MORE INSIGHTS

TODAY, I WANT TO DELVE into the connection between your conscious mind, your subconscious mind (spirit), and your physical body.

When I do prison ministry, I'm not always greeted with a warm reception. I've been heckled by some pretty scary guys! "Your life is easy, white boy!" they shout. "You don't know what it's like!" I used to be intimidated by this, but one day, I just blurted out to someone, "Your best thinking landed you in here!" The crowd was silent for a while, and then a few people started saying "Amen" and "Preach it, brother!" and "That's right, that's right."

When called on it, these guys knew deep down that there was a higher, nobler way of thinking. And some of them still had hope that they could have a much brighter future. The problem simply was that these inmates made choices that conditioned their subconscious minds to believe that bad behavior was the only way to survive.

Conscious Mind = Thinking Mind

The conscious mind is the part of you that thinks and reasons. Your free will lies in this part of your mind, which enables you to choose how you feel about your circumstances and surroundings. Through your conscious mind, you can accept or reject any thought or idea. No external force—person, place, or thing—can cause you to think in a way that you don't choose for yourself.

This is important because it means that you're in charge of all the thoughts and feelings that you accept and that eventually determine the condition of your body and spirit.

Subconscious Mind = Conditioned Mind

The subconscious mind is "godlike." It knows no limits and is the part of your mind that is truly the most magnificent. It is the power center that functions in every cell of your body. When you accept a thought, your subconscious mind takes it and runs with it. As your spirit, it internalizes your thoughts and makes them real, so every thought or word your conscious mind *chooses* to accept, the subconscious mind takes to heart and makes them part of your belief system.

Any thought you *continuously* impress upon your subconscious mind becomes *fixed* in this part of your personality. Fixed ideas, or

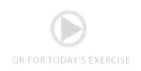

QR FOR TODAY'S EXERCISE

When you accept a thought, your subconscious mind takes it and runs with it.

habits, will continue to express themselves *until they are replaced*. Now, this can be extremely positive or extremely negative depending on the type of thoughts your conscious mind is putting into your subconscious through the thoughts you chose to recognize.

Let's use a fitness example. Your subconscious mind has been imprinted with thoughts on how to view and react to fitness-related topics. You may have lived in a home that didn't see value in fitness, so through the attitudes in your environment, you've been conditioned and domesticated to subconsciously believe that fitness programs and eating right are useless and that you are a victim of your genes. You have relied on what you've learned through repetition, but you are now desperately trying to change. This is where thoughts become imperative to the process of change. It won't happen overnight, and the process of retraining is tedious but worth the effort. Once you begin to alter, adjust, and redirect those thoughts of "fitness is useless" to "a fitness program will benefit me on some level," your actions will slowly begin to change, and you will view fitness in a more positive light.

Fixed ideas, or habits, will continue to express themselves until they are replaced.

The Body = Instrument of the Mind

Most people aren't aware of the power the mind has over the body. Most people perceive the body as the problem because it's the thing they see every day. It's obviously the most visible part of us, but it's also the smallest part in our equation.

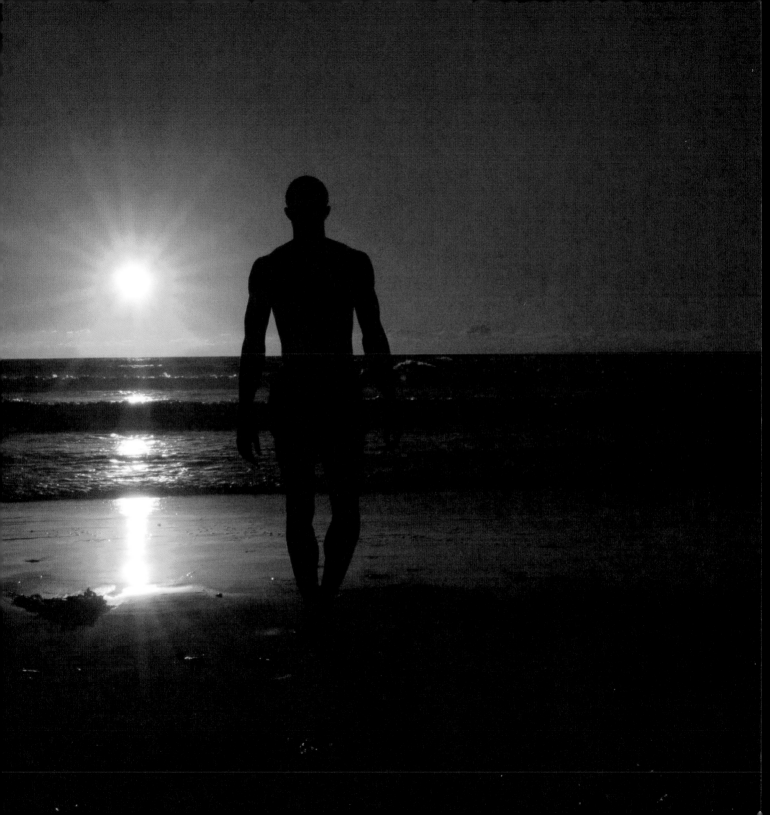

Our beliefs are what affect how we perceive and treat our body...

I like to think of the body as just the house that you live in. And, to a certain extent, you get to decide if you want to live in a clean house or a dirty one, a healthy house or an unhealthy one. Our beliefs are what affect how we perceive and treat our body, just as they affect how we see everything else. If we think we don't have time to exercise, for example, we'll start believing it, and we won't even try to make the time to get in shape. That choice only keeps us accepting more negative thoughts. As the months and years go by and our body becomes unhealthier and weaker, we simply confirm our beliefs and make this belief real to us. We may even convince ourselves that we are trying everything and eating right and that it just isn't working. You can see how easy it is to get stuck in a pattern of bad behavior!

But it's just as simple to set a pattern of good behavior. Having a healthy, functional, vibrant body that's full of life and energy starts with making more and more of the right choices that can properly condition your spirit to move you and begin to replace the habits that keep you feeling bad and accepting of negative thoughts in the first place. For now, start with the little things, like choosing water instead of coffee or soda, and build from there. We'll work on the thoughts you accept and that affect your beliefs later. For now, I want you to start small.

THINK ABOUT THIS!

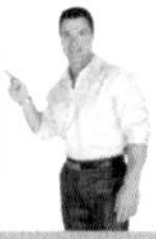

What small choices can you make today that will start to replace negative programming?

_____

_____

_____

_____

_____

_____

_____

_____

_____

_____

_____

THINK YOURSELF A WINNER

THE FOLLOWING POEM SUMMARIZES YESTERDAY'S message—and this entire book for that matter—so read it slowly and repeatedly to allow it to sink into your subconscious mind. I suggest writing it down and placing it where you can see and read it frequently.

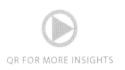

QR FOR MORE INSIGHTS

If you think you are beaten, you are,
If you think you dare not, you don't.
If you like to win, but you think you can't,
It is almost certain you won't.
If you think you'll lose, you're lost,
For out in the world we find,
Success begins with a fellow's will,
It's all in the state of mind.
If you think you are outclassed, you are,

You've got to think high to rise,
You've got to be sure of yourself before
You can ever win a prize.
Life's battles don't always go
To the stronger or faster man.
But soon or late the man who wins,
Is the man who thinks he can.
　　　　　—C. W. Longenecker

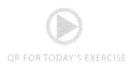

QR FOR TODAY'S EXERCISE

THINK ABOUT THIS!

What areas in your life does this poem make you think about? How can it inspire you?

_____
_____
_____
_____
_____
_____
_____
_____
_____
_____

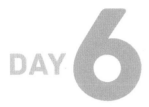

TALK YOURSELF UP!

DAY 6

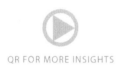

QR FOR MORE INSIGHTS

SOME OF YOU MAY REMEMBER STEVE URKEL saying, "Did I do that?" when he made a stupid comment or did something stupid on the TV show *Family Matters*. Well, I'd like you to start asking yourself that same question whenever you hear negative comments come out of your mouth or when you think a negative thought like any of these:

- It's going to be a bad day.

- I'm so stupid.

- I hate my life.

- Those programs never work for me.

- I'm ugly.

I could go on and on with the negative self-talk that I hear from so many people, myself included from time to time! We all say and think stuff like this without realizing or stopping to think about how much of an impact it really has on how we live our lives and on our minds and bodies. But you know now about the mind-body-spirit connection, so you understand the damage these thoughts can have. You know the self-talk (thoughts) you choose to accept directly affects your self-image (beliefs), and your beliefs affect your life, your health, and your body.

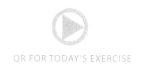
QR FOR TODAY'S EXERCISE

. . . you can change your self-talk . . . and take action to change your beliefs about yourself.

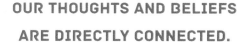

OUR THOUGHTS AND BELIEFS ARE DIRECTLY CONNECTED.

SELF-TALK   (THOUGHTS)

SELF-IMAGE   (BELIEFS)

The good news is that you can change your self-talk, just as you've started to fix your habits, and take action to change your beliefs about yourself. Remember I said we'd work on what thoughts we choose to accept? Well, today's the day.

Actions are the physical steps we take to bring about results and are what we truly need to eliminate negative thoughts.

RESULTS FOLLOW ACTIONS

ACTIONS ➡ EXPECTED RESULTS

. . . when our thoughts and beliefs are out of sync with the results we want, change becomes difficult, if not impossible.

You've already started small positive actions, but now I just want you to start focusing on changing your thoughts and beliefs to help your actions become more effective in your life. When our self-image is strong and our thoughts are positive, our actions can be extremely powerful. But when our thoughts and beliefs are out of sync with the results we want, change becomes difficult, if not impossible. That's why it's important to work on our thoughts and beliefs so we can take the right actions and so those actions have the right results.

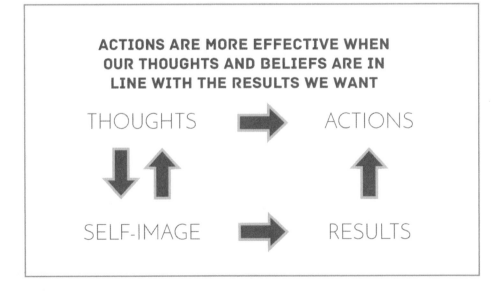

ACTIONS ARE MORE EFFECTIVE WHEN OUR THOUGHTS AND BELIEFS ARE IN LINE WITH THE RESULTS WE WANT

THOUGHTS ➡ ACTIONS

SELF-IMAGE ➡ RESULTS

Throughout the day, write down all your self-talk, good and bad, as you become aware of it and consider how it is affecting what you believe about yourself. Use this to become more aware of what thoughts you choose and allow into your subconscious mind. Then, use that knowledge to stop negative thoughts in their tracks.

THINK ABOUT THIS!

How can you change your thoughts and beliefs for the better?

_____
_____
_____
_____
_____
_____
_____
_____
_____

DAY 7

STOP COMPARING YOURSELF TO OTHERS

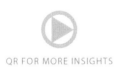

QR FOR MORE INSIGHTS

RADIO TALK SHOW HOST DENNIS PRAGER often shares how his mother used to say something like, "The happiest people I know are the ones I haven't met yet." This means that we all have problems, even the people who seem like they don't.

In our culture, which glorifies physical perfection and sex appeal to a disproportionate degree, this knowledge is really important. It's easy to look at movie stars, models, pro athletes, and other celebrities and think less of ourselves. Instead of drawing inspiration from these people, we end up resenting them, participating in negative self-talk, and feeling insecure. We become involved and engaged with others in an envious way rather than in a healthy connecting way.

I know the most beautifully fit women in the world, but they have the worst self-images I have ever seen. They are constantly looking to someone else or the scale to get edification or something to strive for. When does this end? When will we be happy? Money, fame, weight, material things—these outside things bring us limited joy. At some point, we need to stop looking outside and start turning inside.

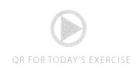

QR FOR TODAY'S EXERCISE

I've been blessed to have a wife who understands and supports my not-so-normal career as a fitness personality. I've traveled the world alone with beautiful models and appeared in magazines, television shows, and movies with more beautiful women, so, needless to say, she's had to deal with her fair share of pressure and insecurity.

The following chapter is her story, taken from my book *Spiritually Fit*:

Doing It for the Right Reasons: The Story of Anita Bartram

Some of the people Clark runs into in his line of work can be pretty superficial, and for some reason they hold me to a higher standard. They have a preconceived notion that I must be this perfect, flawless creature, and I often find myself thinking that I'm supposed to live up to their false standards.

And then there are all the women Clark works with. I admit I have a hard time with that sometimes. Not because I don't trust Clark, but because I tend to compare myself to the "perfect" images these girls convey in their photographs. That can be a lot of pressure!

To top it all off, I seem to be a living example of the scripture that says familiarity breeds contempt. I know Clark's an expert who can get anyone in the best shape possible—I've seen it

The happiest people I know are the ones I haven't met yet.

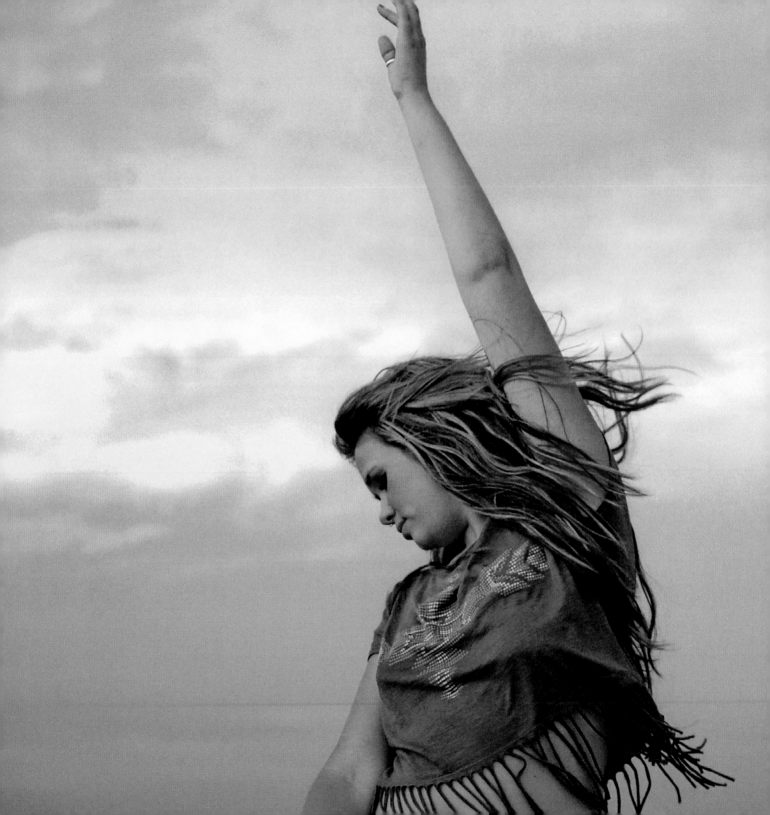

happen countless times with his clients and fans who tell him how he's been an inspiration to them. But I often find myself not wanting advice from him. I guess I just take it too personally. Even if I ask him a question and he innocently says something like "maybe those chips aren't such a great idea," I hear "you're fat and out of shape!"

Clark doesn't put any pressure on me, but I sure put pressure on myself! It's something I've had to work through, and as challenging as it's been it's helped me grow. I'm not out of shape, but I could do better. I may indulge in a snack from time to time (By the way, so does Clark, but don't tell him I told you that!), but I try not to overdo it. And let me tell you, when you're surrounded by people who are paid to stay super-fit all the time, you tend to get a little self-conscious no matter how good a shape you're in!

For me, fitness isn't a profession, but it's important in my life. When I stop comparing myself to others, when I keep things in the right perspective, I find great pleasure and joy in exercise and good nutrition. I exercise and eat right because it feels good, and also because I want to set a good example for my children[…]

I love being married to Clark, and our relationship has stood the test of time because it has many dimensions—physical, mental, and spiritual. I may get frustrated or intimidated by his profession sometimes, but I know that's an illusion that isn't real. Maybe you've had the same pressures from images you've

When I stop comparing myself to others . . . I find great pleasure and joy in exercise and good nutrition.

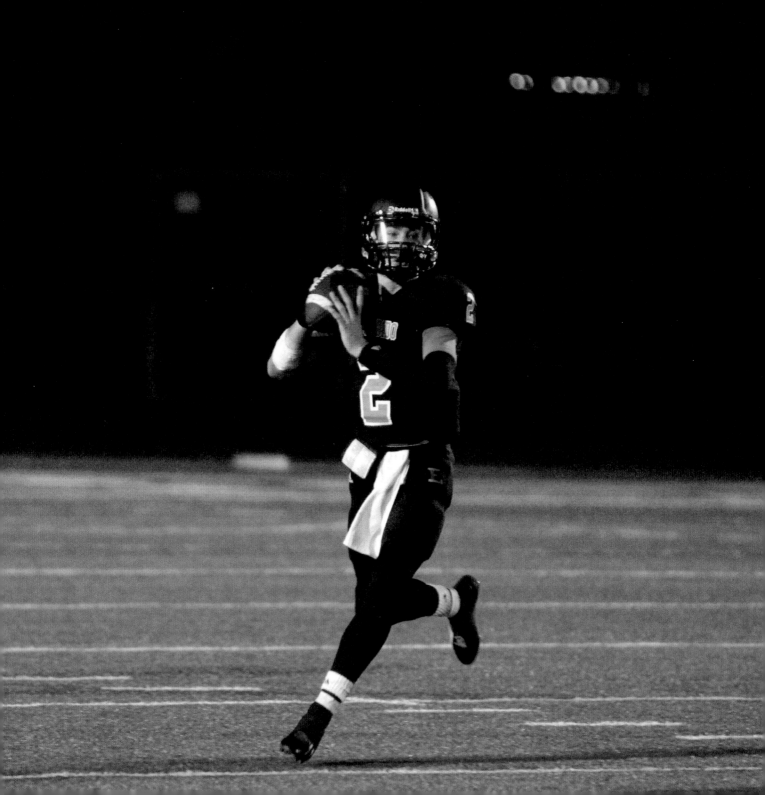

seen on TV or in magazines. Believe me, all those people aren't perfect (I've met a lot of them and they don't even pretend to be!) and if you can relax, try not to be so hard on yourself, and get in shape for the right reasons for you, I think your fitness endeavors will be a lot more fun and a lot easier, too.

Accepting who you are and how special and unique you are is more important than you realize. It's like that saying, "If you're not happy with one dollar, then you won't be happy with a million." Focus on the good things you offer the world, on positive thoughts about yourself, instead of how much better you think other people are, and you'll put yourself on an incredibly rewarding path to success and freedom.

THINK ABOUT THIS!

How have you let the people around you or society at large affect how you see and value yourself? Who do you compare yourself to most often? Are you aware of any challenges they face in their lives? If not, do you really think that they don't have any problems?

_____

_____

_____

_____

_____

_____

REBOOT

DAY 8

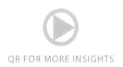

QR FOR MORE INSIGHTS

I **ADMIT THAT I DON'T KNOW** a whole lot about computers. When I have an IT issue, I call my friend Mark. Computers are his thing, not mine, so I've learned to defer to his expertise in all things high tech.

Once I explain to Mark what's going on, the first thing he usually asks me is, "When was the last time you rebooted?" My typical response is, "I dunno." He laughs and tells me to reboot and call him back, and seven out of ten times, it fixes the problem.

My point with this story is that we can usually fix our own life issues when we re-boot our minds. We need to shut down the system, clear it of any bugs, and start it again clean. Our minds are amazing, but just like computers, they need preventive maintenance from time to time.

As we go through life, fragments of places we shouldn't have gone (both on a computer and with ourselves) have been placed in the hard drive, where they wreak havoc on the processor. When we reboot or clean a computer hard drive, one of the processes that happen is "defragging" all the clutter that takes up valuable space, space meant for creating positive outcomes. Rebooting takes us back to a baseline, a foundation where we can work on negative self-talk and ourselves effectively without all the extra noise.

Before we get into the process, one thing to keep in mind is that too often when we run into a problem we yell, break stuff, and cause even more damage. My suggestion is that you reboot your mind and body fast. Don't kick and scream and cause more clutter. Just do it.

Here's how the process of re-booting your mind works, at least as far as I see it:

FIND YOUR PURPOSE

The first thing you need to do is decide what you want to achieve. It all starts with purpose, a decision, a solid WHY. Do you want bigger muscles or a slimmer waist? Do you want to eat better? Do you want to be a more loving spouse? Write it down everything you want to achieve and don't hold back.

When you have your list of goals in front of you, select the two or three that are the most important to you. Write down an affirmation for each of these goals. An affirmation is a simple statement that creates a vivid picture of a goal in your mind, as if it's already been achieved.

Your affirmations should be as specific as possible and should be phrased, as my friend Jon Benson says, so that they "future pace"

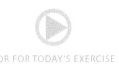

QR FOR TODAY'S EXERCISE

Rebooting takes us back to a baseline, a foundation where we can work on negative self-talk and ourselves effectively without all the extra noise.

"To stay motivated, think about how achieving your goals will impact your entire life."

yourself. A lot of people recommend that you phrase your affirmations in the present tense, but Jon suggests that this shuts down key brain centers that you want to have active when you're making an affirmation. "When you say, 'I am a walrus,'" John says, "your body and your conscious mind know that you're lying." A better solution is to start each affirmation with a more truthful "I'm in the process of ..." or "I'm well on my way to ..." so that your brain believes you, and you can get the results you're after.

To be effective, each one of your affirmations should meet these criteria:

1. Starts with "I'm well on my way to ..." or "I'm in the process of ..."

2. Is short and specific

3. Is positive (The mind doesn't respond to words like "don't," "not," "no," etc.)

4. Includes an action "-ing" word

Here are some examples of fitness affirmations:

- I'm well on my way to wearing size six dresses.

- I'm well on my way to eating only fresh, whole foods.

- I'm well on my way to losing fat and gaining muscle.

- I'm well on my way to walking along the beach without a shirt.

Keep your list of affirmations with you and say each one OUT LOUD as many times a day as you can to help your mind focus on your new reality. As you say each affirmation out loud, create a corresponding visual picture in your mind. See yourself as healthy, fit, attractive, and loving. See yourself with bigger muscles or less fat. See yourself making smart nutrition choices. And always remember to consider how the accomplishment of your specific goals makes you feel. This affirmation exercise is probably the most important thing you can do if you're serious about reaching your goals.

PUT YOUR GOALS IN THE CONTEXT OF YOUR LIFE

At this point, some of you are probably thinking that this is pretty silly stuff. But I promise you, it works!

To stay motivated, think about how achieving your goals will impact your entire life. Think of how much better your relationships with your spouse, your kids, your parents, your friends, and your co-workers will be as you progress toward the positive outcomes you can visualize.

. . . ask yourself what a person who has the goal you want to have would be DOING today.

Getting in shape may seem like a superficial thing, but when you realize how it can impact the way you love your spouse, perform at the office, and play with your kids, it takes on a much deeper meaning.

TURN THOUGHT INTO ACTIONS

I use the "bridge question" to help people take actions that are in alignment with their goals. It's really quite simple and incredibly effective.

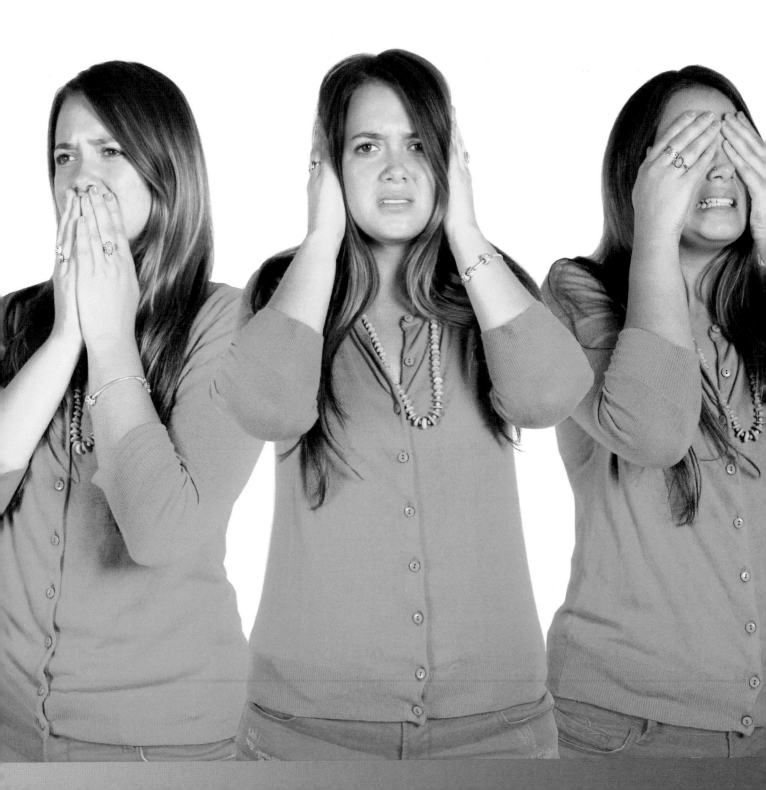

Just ask yourself what a person who has attained your goal would be DOING today. For myself, I ask, "What would a spiritually balanced, physically fit, healthy, God-loving person be doing today? Would he be watching television or going to the gym for an invigorating workout? Would he be stressing out over a family matter or trying to resolve his problems through open communication? Would he be having a soda or a glass of water?" You get the idea.

Try it with everything you do. The person you want to be would definitely be reading this book, so you're already off to a great start! As you do this, be honest with yourself and what's needed in your life. Then, keep this up as long as you think you need to.

PERSISTENCE PAYS OFF

As you do these exercises, chances are that you're going to encounter resistance. You might doubt the power of these exercises and think they won't work. Those around you may think what you're doing is stupid or remind you of your past failures. Try to be persistent even in the face of negative thinking, whether it comes from yourself or others. It took you years to develop negative thought patterns, so it's going to take some time to replace them with positive ones.

...be persistent even in the face of negative thinking, whether it comes from yourself or others.

Throughout this book, I constantly remind you that you're not perfect, and I don't mean that as a criticism. I only say it so that small setbacks don't discourage you and lead to bigger failures. If you expect and accept setbacks and know that someone is with you every step of the way, whether it's a friend or God or whatever deity you believe in, you'll be more likely to regroup and once again move forward toward your goals.

A QUICK REFRESHER: MY THREE MIND EXERCISES FOR HEALTH AND HAPPINESS

I got a little carried away with this chapter and gave you a lot of information to work with today. So here's a quick summary of today's lesson on how to reboot:

Repeat affirmations of your top two or three goals several times out loud daily. This is probably the most important thing you can do to improve your life.

You'll be more motivated when you think about how your success can help you...

Remind yourself that even seemingly superficial goals have deeper meaning in the context of your life and find that context. You'll be more motivated when you think about how your success can help you relate to your family and friends, enhance your career, and better live out the rest of your life.

Use the "bridge question" to ensure you take actions that match your goals. What would a type of person who has the goal you want be DOING?

THINK ABOUT THIS!

Get some 3x5 cards and write your affirmations on them. Then put them everywhere you can see them and say them out loud when you do!

How does the affirmation exercise make you feel? Silly? Nervous? Psyched up? Write down your reactions and think about how you can change them to be more positive if necessary.

_____

_____

_____

_____

_____

_____

_____

_____

_____

MY SEVEN-STEP, GOAL-SETTING BATTLE PLAN

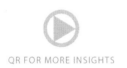

QR FOR MORE INSIGHTS

"In the absence of clearly defined goals, we become strangely loyal to performing daily trivia until ultimately we become enslaved by it."

—Robert Heinlein

MANY PEOPLE TALK ABOUT THE IMPORTANCE of goal setting when it comes to living a fitness lifestyle, but I believe that it's just one step in the overall process. I'm going to give you a very valuable worksheet later in this chapter, but before we get to that, I want to talk about something people often overlook when setting goals: putting your goals in writing.

Committing your goals to a piece of paper or a computer file is one of the best ways to manifest real action. As a permanent record of your intentions, written goals tend to be more thoroughly thought-out, more deeply desired, and more actively worked on. If you're not serious enough to commit your goals to writing, you may as well kiss them goodbye. Life will get busy, you'll get distracted and you'll continue to get the results you're getting now. This is especially true when it comes to eating right, working out, and getting in better shape. If you're going to make a break to greater success, you have to take the time to decide what you want, get 100 percent committed to it, and create a plan to make it happen.

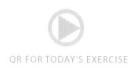

QR FOR TODAY'S EXERCISE

My seven-step goal-setting process will help you think through, clarify, and achieve worthwhile goals. Depending on your current life situation, the goals you choose might be huge, or they might be relatively modest. Ideally, your goals should be aggressive enough to be meaningful, but also realistic enough so you can accomplish them in relatively short order.

> *"Concerning all acts of initiative and creation, there is one elementary truth: that the moment one definitely commits oneself, and then providence moves too. Whatever you can do or dream you can, begin it. Boldness has genius, power, and magic in it. Begin it now."*
> —Johann Wolfgang Von Goethe

Committing your goals to a piece of paper or a computer file is one of the best ways to manifest real action.

START ACHIEVING YOUR GOALS NOW WITH MY SEVEN-STEP, GOAL-SETTING WORKSHEET:

Step 1: List three goals (not two, not four, but three!).

Write down three goals, big or small, that you'd like to accomplish. If appropriate, designate a deadline you will accomplish each one by.

Step 2: Write down a benefit statement for each goal.

What will you get out of achieving those goals? Go deep and think about how achieving your goal will impact your family, friendships, career, health, etc. (This is like when you put your goals in context yesterday.)

Step 3: Identify obstacles.

Every hero has dragons to slay. Sometimes, it's ourselves—we often get in our own way more than anything else. Sometimes, it's other people who would love nothing more than to see you fail because misery loves company. Think about your life and ask yourself what are your obstacles? Write down some of the obstacles you think you might encounter on the way to accomplishing your goals. Write down everything you can think of.

Step 4: Create a strategy.

Here's where you get to think about how you'll overcome each of the obstacles you're about to face. Get creative and write down as many strategies as you can. For example, if you know you stop on the way home from work at a fast food restaurant when you are hungry, have food already prepared that you enjoy or start a journal of what you eat.

Step 5: Recruit your army.

Support from friends, colleagues, associates, experts, and family members is essential for making positive change. It's powerful for two reasons. First of all, going public with your plan to the people in your life makes it more difficult to blow it off. Secondly, getting support helps you stay focused and disciplined. A wise man used to tell me, "You're only committed to what you confess." Write down the people who will help keep you accountable and support you in your efforts.

If you're going to make a break to greater success, you have to take the time to decide what you want, get 100 percent committed to it, and create a plan to make it happen.

Step 6: Set up a victory party.

How will you reward yourself when you achieve your goals? And, just as important, what will happen if you don't achieve your goals?

The inner satisfaction of accomplishing a difficult task is sometimes the single greatest reward. But it's also motivating to establish an external reward system, an incentive you give to yourself such as a vacation or some new clothing. If one of your goals is an ongoing one, like making ten sales contacts per day or exercising five times per week, then pick a random date (one month from now, ninety days from now, etc.) to celebrate your progress.

Step 7: Pick the day you declare war.

The final step is committing to an official start date for each of your goals. Make sure you're prepared … but don't delay!

The inner satisfaction of accomplishing a difficult task is sometimes the single greatest reward. But it's also motivating to establish an external reward system...

Failure to plan is planning to fail. Why haven't you set goals and focused on them? Use your answer to help you with Step 3 of your battle plan, the one about identifying obstacles.

THINK ABOUT THIS!

_____

_____

_____

_____

_____

DAY 10

WHAT IS YOUR WHY?

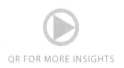

QR FOR MORE INSIGHTS

AS I'VE HINTED AT ALREADY, too often in life we do things for the wrong reasons, especially in the area of fitness. Motives like "I want to look good at my high school reunion to make everyone jealous" will never lead to lasting results. Other vain and superficial reasons—like "I want a six-pack" or "I want to look hot in a bikini"—usually aren't good enough to adopt a fitness lifestyle with vigor and tenacity for very long.

To put your goals in the proper context, like we've already done on a couple of occasions in this mental journey, you must drill deeper and enter an emotional space that you may not have explored for a long time.

This section may seem repetitive or meaningless or extremely difficult. No matter how it makes you feel, give it a try and do your best to open yourself up to the process of self-discovery. You may be surprised by what happens. You may experience emotions that have been buried beneath the protective layers of justification and forget-fulness for years.

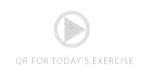

QR FOR TODAY'S EXERCISE

Here's what I suggest you do to get to your true reason for doing something, your particular "why." Start with a desire and then drill it down at least four or five levels deep, like the following example:

"I want to get in shape."

Why?

"Because I want to look better in a bathing suit."

Why?

"Because I want my spouse to be attracted to me!"

Why?

"Because I feel like we've been growing apart."

Why?

"Because my spouse flirts with other people, and I'm feeling jealous."

(Okay, now we're getting somewhere.) Why?

"Because I think my spouse is attracted to other people instead of me. I'm overweight, and I've been grumpy every day because I hate the way I look."

To put your goals in the proper context . . . you must drill deeper and enter an emotional space that you may not have explored for a long time.

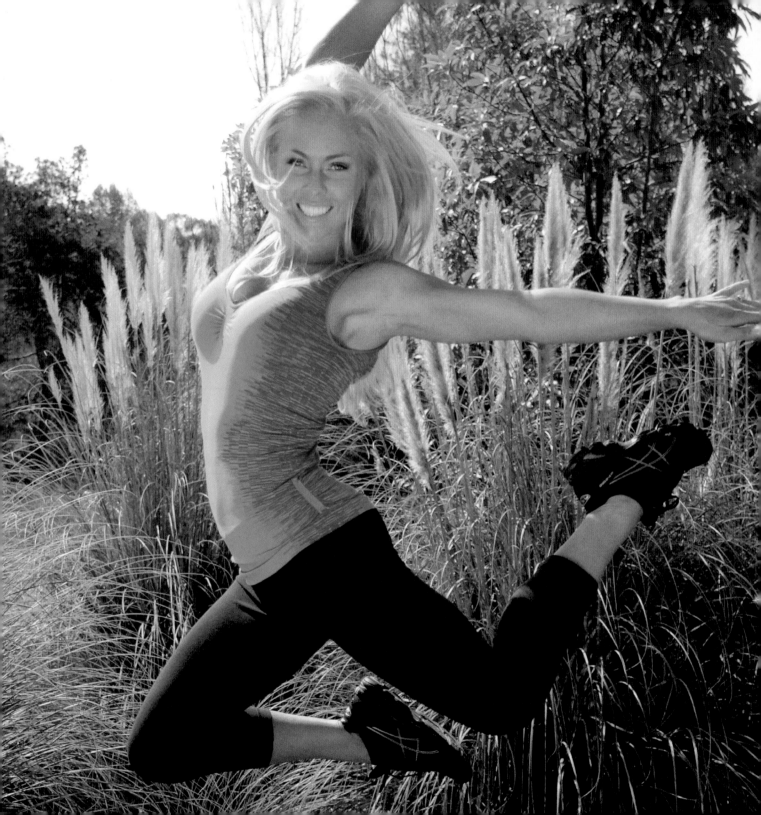

See where I'm going with this? This type of emotional exercise has brought up some deep things with my clients. Once you discover your true motivations for improving your life, your goals will become essential to your happiness instead of things that would simply be nice to have. It becomes an emotional journey. You'll take your goals more seriously and work harder to get the results you're after.

THINK ABOUT THIS!

Take the three goals you listed yesterday and delve deeper into your "why" for each one. Did what you found surprise you?

11

KNOW THE DIFFERENCE BETWEEN COMMITMENT AND EXCITEMENT

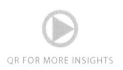

QR FOR MORE INSIGHTS

I'VE BEEN A COACH ON many levels for the past twenty-five years, and I've seen people mistake excitement for commitment too many times.

Let's create a scenario here: A team is gathered together before the big game. The team captain steps into the huddle and gives a motivational speech to his teammates. They start jumping up and down, put their hands in the middle, say their team mantra, and rush the field for the opening kickoff.

They kick to the opposing team, and things suddenly break down. A few guys miss a tackle while others get knocked flat on their backs. The runner gracefully maneuvers his way through all eleven players and hits the promised land—TOUCHDOWN! The teammates start placing blame on each other, losing their excitement.

This has happened thousands of times, and it will continue to happen—not just on the football field, but also everywhere people let excitement drive them instead of commitment.

A way around this is to focus on facts instead of feelings. One of my mentors shared an illustration of a train with me, to demonstrate how we should drive our thoughts and actions. In the illustrations below, you'll see two trains. We all know that the engine at the front of the train is the power source that pulls the rest of the cars.

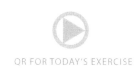

QR FOR TODAY'S EXERCISE

RIGHT WAY

EMOTION 🚃 FEELING 🚂 FACT

WRONG WAY

FACT 🚃 EMOTION 🚂 FEELING

Most people let emotions drive the train of their lives when it should really be facts that have all the power. Emotions change and can take you on a crazy rollercoaster ride. Facts don't change and can help you make steady progress.

So let's recreate our football scenario in light of this information. The beginning of the game starts the same way—the motivation speech,

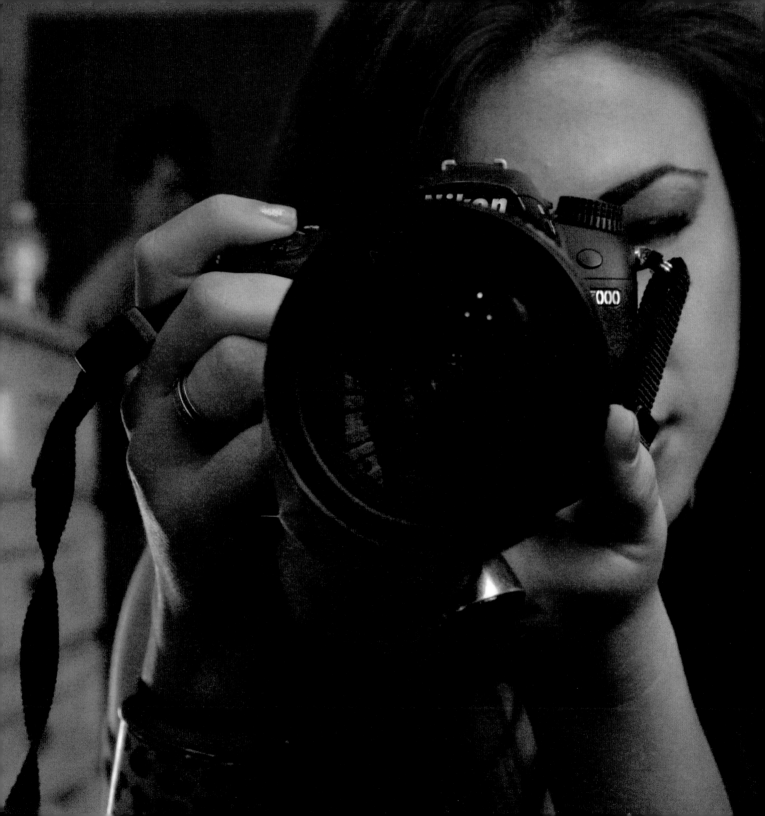

the kick to the opposing team, the missed tackles. Again, the opposing runner gracefully maneuvers his way through all eleven players and hits the promised land—TOUCHDOWN!

This time, the team captain refocuses the attention of his teammates: "Okay, guys, this is what we trained for. This is why we lift all those weights, practice on Saturdays, and sweat our butts off in the heat of the summer. We have trained for this, and we know how to do it. Here's the play: 291, Smoke Jet Thirty-Three, Streak on Two … Let's go out there and do what we've been coached to do on every play. Regardless of what happens, we'll be all right. We can do this!"

This kind of commitment requires an unemotional, objective look at whatever the facts may be, and it takes a lot of practice. Sometimes you win and sometimes you lose, but when you face a setback you always have the CHOICE to control how you approach the next play, step, meal, conversation, or thought in your head!

Most people let emotions drive the train of their lives when it should really be facts that have all the power.

THINK ABOUT THIS!

What's driving your train? What situations push your emotional buttons? Do you only show commitment when things are going well? How can you maintain your commitment when the excitement diminishes?

_____

_____

_____

_____

12

MAKE CHOICES THAT WILL SATISFY YOU LATER

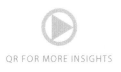

QR FOR MORE INSIGHTS

OFTEN THE DIFFERENCE BETWEEN PEOPLE who do and people who don't is just a decision. I've heard it said, and it's true, that "The decisions you make today will determine the circumstances of the rest of your life." So let's improve your decision-making power!

How many times in life have you made a decision, knowing all along that the outcome would leave you feeling empty, guilty, or ashamed? I've done it on more occasions than I'd like to admit.

Every day, we're presented with two choices—the right one and the wrong one. It's that simple. Think about food, for example. How many times have you eaten something that you know will make you feel guilty later, just because it tastes good now? Convenience, cost, availability, and enjoyment all come into play when we make a wrong choice by hitting the drive-thru. Laziness, procrastination, and rationalizing are all excuses when it comes to your fitness choices; and ignorance, instant gratification, and "keeping up with the Jones'" are some of the reasons we get into financial trouble.

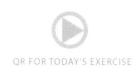

There are restaurants out there that offer "guilt-free" options on the menu, but in most cases, you're on your own and have to weigh consequences of your pleasure-seeking ways. I don't know of anyone who has cheated on a diet who didn't feel horrible about it later. Problem being, people think of what will satisfy them at that moment, not how they feel when they will want to puke after bingeing on food. Our whole world is about instant gratification, but our society has it all backward and has messed many of us up. It is my intention to turn things inside out. I want you to start making choices based on *delayed* gratification.

All of the bad *decisions* I've mentioned could have been easily counteracted by the opposite choice:

- Budgeting and understanding what you truly need can help keep you out of debt.

- Being prepared can circumvent convenience when it comes to food choices.

- Esteeming others above yourself will keep you from cheating.

- Deciding once and for all that a fitness lifestyle is required for a productive life will overcome laziness and procrastination.

Our whole world is about instant gratification . . . I want you to start making choices based on delayed gratification.

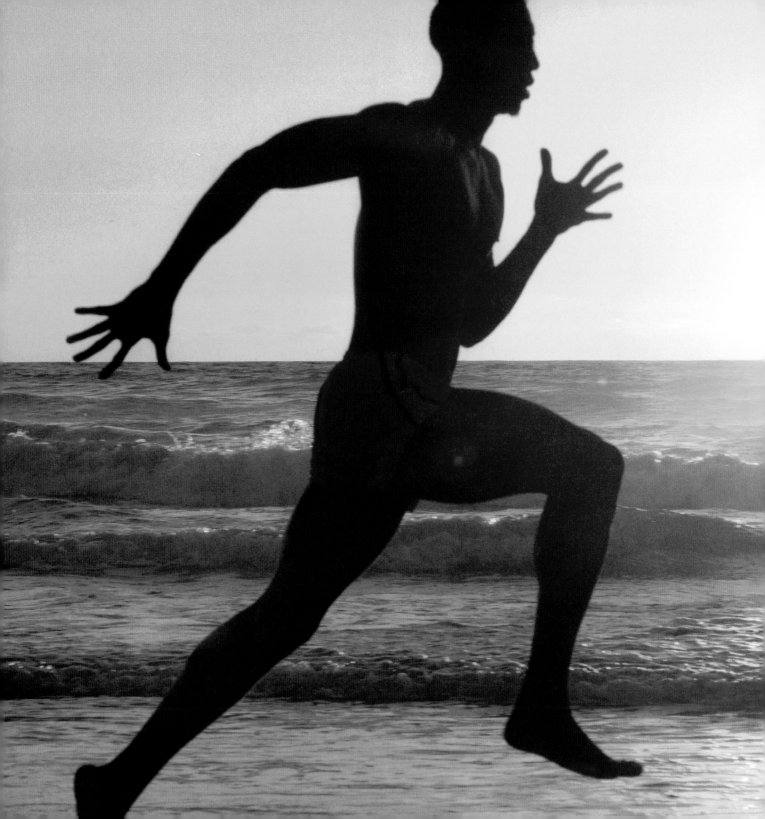

When you understand the true power that lies in the results of your positive decisions, making the right choices becomes a much easier process. Throughout the day today, I want you to really get it into your head that everything you do is a CHOICE and that your CHOICES determine your future satisfaction. But before you make any choices today, think about the long-term consequences and see if that changes your mind. Try to think past the immediate gratification and anticipate how you'll feel tomorrow, next week, next month, or next year after you make a certain choice.

THINK ABOUT THIS!

Look up the word "choice" in a thesaurus and notice all the synonyms. Write down the ones that seem empowering to you. Remember these throughout the day.

_____

_____

_____

_____

_____

_____

_____

13

BE PATIENT WITH YOURSELF

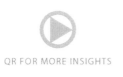

DO YOURSELF A FAVOR: as you start making better choices, don't beat yourself up every time you make a bad choice (I did say I would remind you that you aren't perfect throughout the book.). Just come to terms with your bad choice and move on to better decisions.

Be patient with yourself. I remember once trying to figure out some fitness materials that were way over my head at the time. I was getting very frustrated because I just couldn't get it. I decided to pick up the phone and call the author, and much to my surprise, he answered. When I told him that I was having trouble understanding the material, his immediate response was, "Just relax, Clark. We learn in layers." That told me that I wasn't as stupid as I thought I was and made me feel more confident that one day I'd get a fuller under-standing of what I was trying to learn. And sure enough, about three months later, the information suddenly made sense as I was working with a personal training client. The new context helped me achieve a new "layer" of understanding.

And it's no different with what we're trying to accomplish here. You are 100 percent capable of making the right decisions and achieving success in every area of your life—faith, finances, family, and fitness. It just might take time and effort and a few slip-ups along the way. That's part of it.

Results come to different people at different times as long as they avoid frustration and consistently move toward their desired goals. More simply stated, be consistent and let the results come when they come, not when you want them to. Focus more on the process of making better choices than the outcome, and you'll get your desired results in due time.

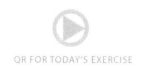

QR FOR TODAY'S EXERCISE

THINK ABOUT THIS!

Have you made the right decisions in your life? If not, are you willing to make better ones to get the things you want out of life?

_____

_____

_____

_____

_____

_____

_____

14

DISCOVER WHY PRACTICE DOESN'T MAKE PERFECT

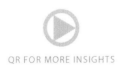

QR FOR MORE INSIGHTS

I'VE HEARD THE SAYING "PRACTICE** makes perfect" thrown around for years, and I just don't think it's completely true.

Consider this: you're in elementary school, and you're getting your first lessons on addition and subtraction. Your assignment is to go home and practice 2+2=4. But what if you get your wires crossed and start practicing 2+2=5? Does that change the fact that 2+2=4? Does it help you learn what 2+2 equals? Of course not! If you practice the wrong things, you won't get perfect. Not even close. And you're not going to get different results either.

In my opinion, the saying should really be that perfect practice makes you better. The point is that great results are possible in all areas of life as long as you are using an approach that works for you. This may take some searching, and the same approach may not work forever, but finding the right one is necessary for growth.

For example, maybe you've been exercising regularly but aren't getting stronger or losing weight. It could be because you're on the wrong fitness program or because you aren't also eating right or getting enough rest. Or it could be because the trainer you hired isn't motivating or because you've hit a plateau, and what worked for you in the first three months doesn't work now. We all hit plateaus, myself included. It's vital we get creative with a new practice plan and are willing to change when needed. For example, I was tired of working out, so I joined another gym—fresh environment, fresh attitude.

There are a million different variables, and you have to constantly refine your practice if you want to continually improve and make sure it's perfectly what you need to get the result you strive for. We MUST evolve. Otherwise, we die. We don't even stagnate. That's not possible. If we don't move forward, we always decline.

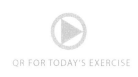

QR FOR TODAY'S EXERCISE

Are you practicing something without getting results? If so, what changes can you make to practice more perfectly?

THINK ABOUT THIS!

_____

_____

_____

_____

_____

DAY 15 — GET A CHANGE OF SCENERY

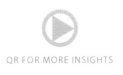

QR FOR MORE INSIGHTS

SEVERAL YEARS AGO, I STARTED doing some brainstorming sessions with a dear friend of mine. He was in L.A. and I was in San Diego, about a two-hour drive for either one of us. He'd always ask me to drive up to see him, and this started to tick me off a little bit. I used to think, *"Why doesn't he ever come to my house?"*

Well, I figured it out one time when I arrived at our destination. You see, he'd always pick a very high-end hotel and we'd meet in the lobby. At first, I was very uncomfortable with this. I fought it. "This isn't me," I'd protest. "I don't belong here—look at all these pretentious people walking around!" I was hating on these people and couldn't see myself in their position.

My friend and I would sit and talk in these extravagant places, and eventually I began to accept the fact that it was okay to have abundance. Many of the people who stayed at these resorts probably worked really hard for it. I started to loosen up and allowed my mind to expand. I became very productive as a result of these brainstorming sessions, and that made the two-hour drive worth it.

You're probably wondering how this relates to you and your desire to grow mentally, emotionally, and physically. Well, what I'm suggesting is that you consider getting a change of scenery at least once a month. Ruts are slow-dug graves. We need to break out of the norm and enjoy something different even if it's just an overnight stay in a nice hotel room. If you sit in your house every day, take the same drive to work, eat the same foods, watch the same shows, and never engage a strange person, life can suck fast and you never expand your mind beyond what you already have and know.

So get a fresh outlook. See things you've never seen. Smell smells you've never smelled. Eat food you've never tried. Find a high-end hotel in your area and just spend some time in the lobby like I did. You could meet a friend or a mentor, read a chapter of this book and reflect for an hour, or just watch the parade of people go by. You never know what might happen, who you might meet, or how it could expand your worldview and inspire you.

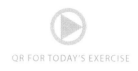

QR FOR TODAY'S EXERCISE

THINK ABOUT THIS!

Write a list of places you could go for your change of scenery. Pick one to go to today and write down your thoughts. Were you uncomfortable? Inspired? Both?

_____

_____

_____

_____

DAY 16

IS THE "EMOTIONAL SNIPER" STALKING YOU?

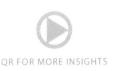

QR FOR MORE INSIGHTS

NOW THAT YOU'RE HALFWAY THROUGH this thirty-day program, I want to double check that you're really on the right track—that your goals are aligned with your core values.

Recently, I was watching a reality show that's popular among kids today. One of the stars chose to leave the program because of his anxiety. In the interest of full disclosure, I'll confess that I've watched this show long enough to know the whole backstory, so I feel I may have identified the "root" of this young man's anxiousness.

Throughout the different episodes, you see how this guy grew up in a solid, very close-knit Italian family with some deep core values. He was a self-admitted "mama's boy," and the event that caused his breakdown was seeing his mother for the first time after a few months of being away. He began to cry and said, "I'm not sure if I should be happy or sad."

I believe that when he saw his mother, he realized that she had been watching him act out on national television for years. He couldn't take the guilt and the pain he caused his mother, and he walked away from fame, money, and all the other trappings of his dream of supposed success.

This guilt can be a good thing. Society has made us think backward in many cases, and our definition of guilt and how we are conditioned to respond to it has made us see guilt wrong. We run from it when we actually need to embrace it. We feel like we need to avoid guilt in order to overcome it and prevent it from ruining our lives, but guilt is our friend, not our enemy. Guilt is there for a specific reason. It's an indicator light on the dashboard of life that says something ain't right and tells you that you better check yourself before you breakdown.

In my view, guilt works like an emotional sniper. If you know anything about the military, you probably know that snipers are taught to take as long as they need to set themselves up in a well-hidden position and take out their targets. Guilt works in much the same way. It sits there for as long as it needs to before going in for the kill. If we act in ways that aren't true to who we are

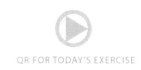

QR FOR TODAY'S EXERCISE

If you're not true to yourself, even achieving your goals can be a defeat instead of a victory.

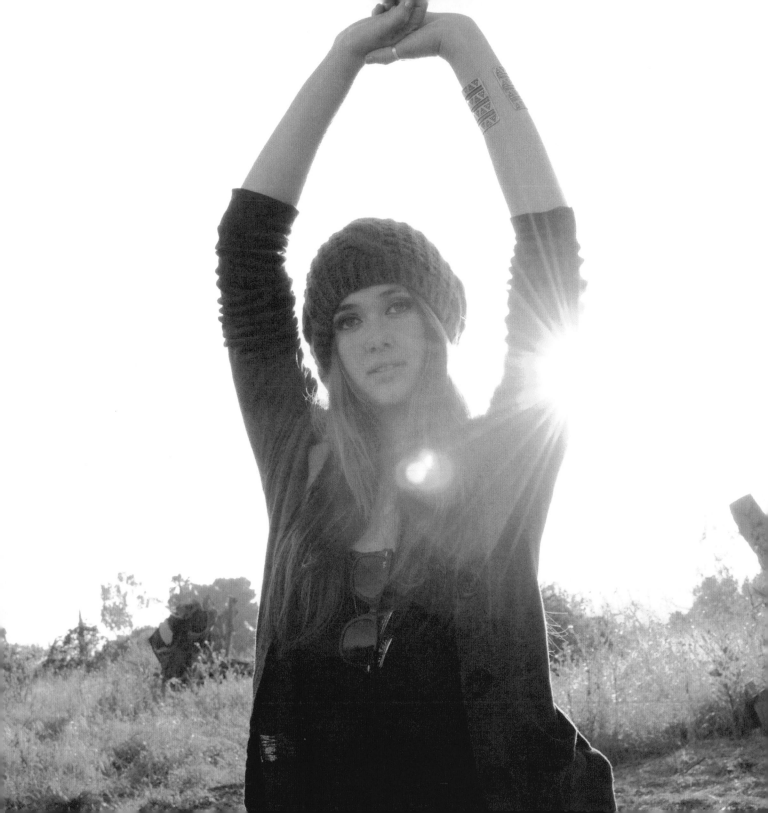

at the core and continue to do so, guilt slowly and steadily creeps into position and takes us out. If you're not true to yourself, even achieving your goals can be a defeat instead of a victory.

That's why it's so important to evaluate your goals, listen to any guilt you have, and make sure you're doing things for the right reasons.

THINK ABOUT THIS!

Is there anything in the back of your mind telling you that your goals aren't aligned with your core values? How can you make adjustments before the emotional sniper takes you out?

_____

_____

_____

_____

_____

_____

_____

_____

_____

_____

_____

EXPAND YOUR SOCIAL NETWORK

YEARS AGO, I DECIDED THAT I was going to say hi to at least five people I didn't know each day—you know, the kinds of people you pass by on the street, share an elevator with, sit next to in a coffee shop.

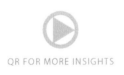

QR FOR MORE INSIGHTS

I was absolutely shocked by the responses I got. Most people returned the greeting, but some people seemed to get downright offended! Other people opened up and had really amazing conversations with me. I found that I feel more fulfilled when I actually engage in meaningful exchanges with others.

Human contact is good for the mind, body, and soul in many different ways. Now, I'm no scientist, and I don't even play one on TV; but I do know our bodies have cascades of hormones that are either released or suppressed by some beautiful process of nature, the creator, God, the Universe, or however you describe it. I know I really like it when someone says hello to me or gives me a random compliment or politely engages me in conversation, and I suspect you're the same way. It's just a nice feeling to make contact with another person.

Life is meant to be interactive and integrative like exercise should be. With exercise, our bodies respond best with workouts that are integrative in nature, meaning exercises that use different body parts together in unison and combine the different functions for an overall purpose of progress and productivity. In life, we are meant to integrate and work with others to create the same positive outcome, to become better by interacting in unison.

I know this from personal experiences. Just today, in the gym, I met a gentleman who enriched my life after a ten-minute conversation. We had an enjoyable chat, and he also has connections that I need at a crossroads in my life. If I hadn't said anything to Jack, I would have missed meeting a great man with a great attitude and great connections that have given me excitement and encouragement to write this today (right in the midst of a big turning point in my own life).

Through engaging with new people daily, even the people who may rub us the wrong way, we can enrich our life and take our mind and body places we could never go by ourselves. Interacting with the people we randomly encounter or helping them opens our eyes to greater possibilities in life and can inspire us to be the best we can be. There are gifts passing you and me every single day, and the only way we can see what they are is by opening them—all with just one word: hello.

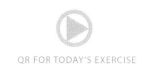

QR FOR TODAY'S EXERCISE

Human contact is good for the mind, body, and soul in many different ways.

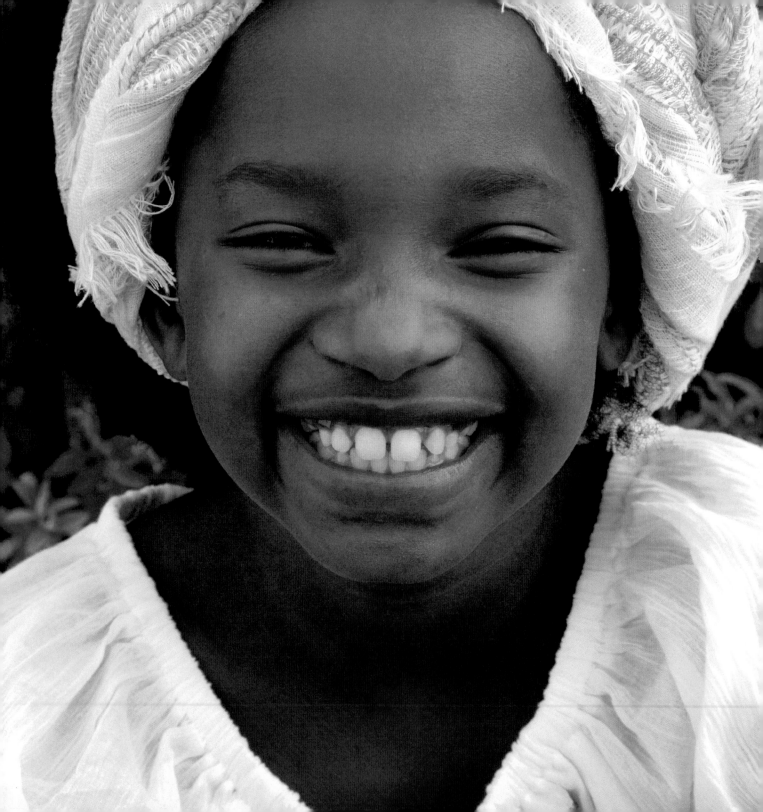

Please do yourself a favor and at least find out if what I'm saying is true. I could go on and on with theory, personal stories, and rhetoric, but YOU must experience it for yourself to see if it is worth your time or not. So try to engage at least five people today in a way that you would like to be engaged. It will certainly be interesting and, hopefully, fun and rewarding.

THINK ABOUT THIS!

Is saying hi to people easy or difficult for you? Do you recall any friendships you have that started with a simple "hello"? Are there any times in your life when you wished you had engaged a stranger in conversation? Does the admonition "Don't talk to strangers," prevent you from making any contact with people?

_____

_____

_____

_____

_____

_____

_____

_____

_____

_____

18

START AND END EACH DAY WITH INTENTION

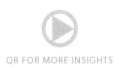

RECENTLY, I'VE BECOME VERY DELIBERATE about what goes into my mind when I wake up in the morning and just before I go to sleep. These days, I especially like the messages of Joyce Meyer, a motivational and inspirational speaker whose ministry focuses on changing your life for the good and who has made a tremendous difference in my approach to life. In general, I believe that programming your brain with positive thoughts at the beginning and end of each day can have a huge impact on how successful we can become.

Most of us just click on the TV or the radio at night and in the morning without even thinking about the negative information coming our way from the news, crime shows, reality TV, and the like. Now, you may be thinking, "It's just the news, and I need to see the weather for the day." Or, "That's my favorite show. It's not that bad."

Well, how important is it for you to be mentally strong? How badly do you want to master your thoughts, feelings, and emotions? How deeply do you desire your goals? Our mind is only programmed by the input we give it, so if your mind starts the day with "Ten were killed today in a massive fire," and ends with "The economy is the poorest it's ever been," and you sprinkle some gossip, bad eating, a lack of exercise, and an argument during the middle of the day, what do you expect to be spit out of the hard drive of your mind? Negativity. That's why exercise is vital, why getting someplace new helps, and why shutting off the TV or changing the channel to something enlightening and positive will be the remedy to turn things around.

Just try this for a month and see what happens. Every day before you go to bed, watch, listen to, or read something positive. And do the same thing when you wake up in the morning. Now, you should be doing this already with this book! If you're not, start now and keep at it for the remaining eleven days. And when you're done, check out Joyce Meyer or other people who can keep you motivated and inspired, and fill the time after you wake up and before you go to bed with those positive messages. Get your news or entertainment fix in the middle of the day and save the beginning and end for more uplifting, positive programming.

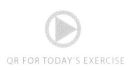

QR FOR TODAY'S EXERCISE

THINK ABOUT THIS!

What occupies your mind in the morning and at night? In addition to this book, what other materials can you read, watch, or listen to that will help motivate you to reach your goals?

_____

_____

_____

_____

_____

DAY 19

APPLY THE RIGHT PRESSURE TO AVOID TOXIC SITUATIONS

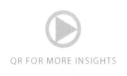

QR FOR MORE INSIGHTS

I'M A PRETTY POSITIVE GUY. You can usually count on me for an encouraging word, and you can trust that I'll do my best to avoid backstabbing and gossip. I'm not perfect, but I try.

Over the past twenty years or so, I've pretty much worked for myself. This has kept me somewhat isolated from the traps and chaos of the corporate world—until recently. Now, I often find myself operating within an environment that includes lots of different personalities, and I've learned very quickly that people love to suck you into whatever particular mess they're going through. I got caught up in a particularly bad situation and learned the hard way how easy it is for others to draw us in. Sometimes it's instantaneous, but other times we don't even notice it until we're up to our eyeballs in the muck.

You don't need nor want that negativity in your life. When you gossip or "return fire" to those who are gossiping and slandering you, you lower yourself, distract yourself from every goal you have, set a bad example, and waste valuable energy on negativity. We either want to move forward or we don't, and gossip will never allow you to move ahead. After all, chances are, right down the hall from your gossip session or in the next cubical over, the gossip is about you. Focus on positivity.

So how can we avoid this negativity? I found the answer when I was showing a group of inmates how strong I was. I used to travel the world ministering in prisons doing "feats of strength." I'd tear phone books, break baseball bats, bend horseshoes, and all kinds of attention- grabbing stunts, all in an attempt to drive home inspiring messages.

One of my favorite feats to perform was the hardest one of all: blowing up an old-fashioned hot water bottle until it burst. This seemed to get people the most engaged—mostly because it was dangerous! At times, I'd lose my hearing in one ear for a while, or the exploding rubber would hit me in the face or whip into a body part I don't care to mention.

One time, I was right in the middle of this stunt in front of about a thousand people, and I just wanted to give up and quit. But my pride wouldn't let me, so I just kept pushing as hard as I could. I knew that eventually the bottle would have to explode.

When the darn thing finally burst, I caught my breath and said to the crowd, "You just sat here and saw me struggling to blow this thing up. And while I was doing it, I had a pretty powerful thought that applies to all of our lives. Are you ready for it? The only way I'm going to be successful doing this is to make the pressure on the inside greater than the pressure on the outside!"

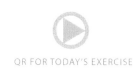

QR FOR TODAY'S EXERCISE

When you gossip or "return fire" to those who are gossiping and slandering you, you lower yourself, distract yourself from every goal you have, set a bad example, and waste valuable energy on negativity.

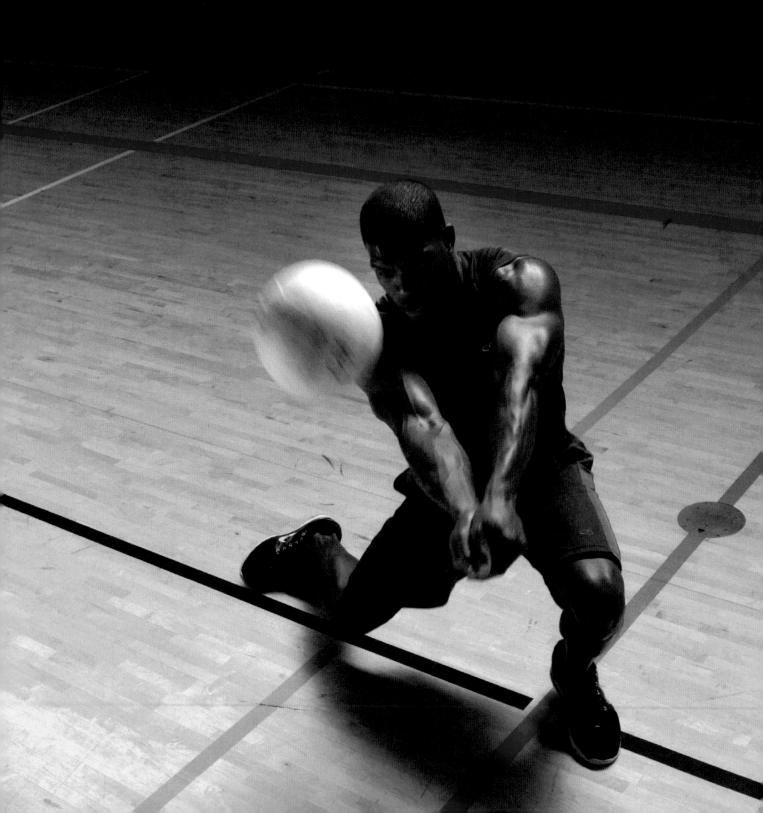

Think about that for a second or an hour or all day—however long it takes for the idea to sink into your soul. The pressure on the inside must be greater than the pressure on the outside! Think about that the next time someone talks trash about someone in the office, especially if it's a person you don't necessarily care for. Is the pressure to get involved in that conversation greater than the knowledge within you that gossip amounts to nothing good at all?

If so, you're in danger of getting involved with miserable people and becoming miserable yourself. So you have to make sure that the pressure within is greater than the external pressure you're getting from your colleagues, friends, or family members. Just think of the hot water bottle the next time someone wants to bring you into a toxic situation!

The pressure on the inside must be greater than the pressure on the outside!

THINK ABOUT THIS!

How often do you engage in negative talk? How do you feel afterward? Do you think people who talk trash or gossip with you do the same about you when you're not around? How can you make sure the pressure on the inside is greater than the pressure on the outside?

_____

_____

_____

_____

_____

_____

_____

20 LOVE YOURSELF

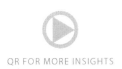

QR FOR MORE INSIGHTS

IF YOU HAD TO DESCRIBE YOURSELF to me right now, what would you say? I know what I'd say about me—I often tell people, "I love me … I'm awesome!" And I'm 100 percent serious. I say that to people for two reasons: one, it's true. I think that—not in a narcissistic, self-centered way, but in a healthy, wholesome way. My love and respect for myself is grounded in my understanding of who I am in God. It certainly isn't because I think I'm better than anyone else. I love being me, I love what I can do for people, and I'm the most awesome person I know. That's what I believe and CHOOSE to repeat in my head. The other reason is that I love the responses I get from people when I say it—positive and negative—and I think it tells me a lot about how people think of themselves.

What was your reaction? Do you wish you could think the same way I do? Or do you think I'm just full of myself? If you want to think the same way about your awesome self, following this daily program and reading this chapter should get you there fairly quickly. If you think there is something wrong with what I said, then your head is probably in the wrong space right now, and I want you to really listen to what I'm about to say. At the beginning of the book, I mentioned that I lost my confidence and that was the reason I wrote the book. Well that lack of confidence also brought some doubt and some self-loathing and ultimately made me focus on the things that I didn't necessarily like about myself. I started seeing my height as something negative. I'm 5'8", and that has bothered me at times. I found myself thinking random fearful thoughts that had me believing I was losing my mind. I could go on and on, but what I want you to understand is that I am also guilty of finding things about myself that I don't necessarily like or appreciate, even though I bragged earlier of how awesome I think I am.

But after going through my own journey, I deeply believe that there's absolutely nothing wrong with loving yourself. Actually, I think it's what God, the Creator, the Higher Power, the Universe, or whatever you want to call it wants you to do; and you need to see that. Loving yourself just makes life that much easier on every single level. People who are self-loathing and have negative beliefs of themselves have a hard time believing they deserve anything good, fitness or otherwise. You saw earlier how my low self-esteem was harmful to me. I lost contracts. Then, the insecurity with my height had me avoiding auditions because I thought casting directors would think I was too

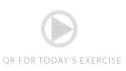

QR FOR TODAY'S EXERCISE

short when, truth be told, I've landed jobs where the character was supposed to be 6'3". My headspace was holding me back before, as yours is. You need to open yourself up to the advantages of loving yourself because, until we get you to that place, it's going to be more difficult for you to consistently think positively about the circumstances and situations you encounter in your life.

Here's a simple exercise for you to start right now, regardless of your headspace. Make a list like the one below:

You need to open yourself up to the advantages of loving yourself because, until we get you to that place, it's going to be more difficult for you to consistently think positively about the circumstances and situations you encounter in your life.

THINGS I LOVE ABOUT MYSELF	THINGS ABOUT MYSELF I CAN LOVE MORE

Notice that I didn't make a column that says "Things I Hate about Myself." That's not even something we're going to entertain. Let's just stay focused on the great things about you and the things about yourself that can become even greater. Deal? Okay then, get started now and continue to work on it all day!

As you go forward, continue to work on loving yourself. Remember to be excellent with you words! Remember that words are powerful—the ones spoken to you by yourself and the words you speak to others. As you may remember from earlier in this book, what you say to yourself is what you allow to become your beliefs and your self-image. You've already written down your negative self-talk and become aware of what you say to yourself. Now, if you haven't already, it's time to take the next step. Just simply stop telling yourself anything you don't see value in about yourself. Is it easy? No, not always, but it is worth it, and it does gets results. Your words and thoughts are vital to your success in every aspect of your life, and you must get them under control now. If you are excellent with your words, you will be excellent in your life, and it will be worth every bit of effort required.

If you are excellent with your words, you will be excellent in your life, and it will be worth every bit of effort required.

Write down how you currently see yourself in one simple sentence. Is it positive, negative or neutral? Has your opinion of yourself limited your enjoyment of life in any way?

THINK ABOUT THIS!

_____

_____

_____

_____

_____

DAY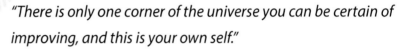

BE THE BEST YOU THAT YOU CAN BE

"There is only one corner of the universe you can be certain of improving, and this is your own self."

—Aldous Huxley

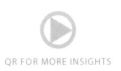

QR FOR MORE INSIGHTS

I HAVE TO SHARE THE story of the middle-aged woman I met on the set of my television show *American Health & Fitness*. I can't remember her name, but how she looked and our conversation will remain embedded in my mind forever.

I walked into the wardrobe trailer where she was preparing her lunch. The smell and the color of the food drew me in. Plus I was probably hungry and wanted some. She was preparing fresh vegetables, a chicken breast, and brown rice. I walked up to her and said, "Wow, what a great lunch!"

Without any hesitation, she looked right at me and said, *"This is the body God gave me, and I'm going to live in it healthy!"* That was, and still is, one of the most powerful statements I've ever heard come out of someone's mouth. She stood 4'11" and weighed at least 200 pounds. And even though she knew she would never be a supermodel, she valued who she was and the body she had. Her self-image was incredibly strong when she could have easily thrown in the towel and said, "Screw it, I'm just going to eat crap because I'm going to be fat anyway." This woman made a conscious decision to live healthy in the body she had. And that's advice all of us should be following.

To me, this and yesterday's chapter could be the most valuable lessons in this entire book! Why? Well, self-love is critical on so many levels. It's the first step in any fitness program. It's a vital step in any personal development process. It's so valuable in parenting effectively and being a great spouse and co-worker. Many people shut down part of who they are by not accepting how they look. I see so many people who rob the world of the value they bring as an individual because they feel they don't measure up to society's standards or they want to look like they did twenty years ago. If you don't love yourself, then on some level, you are holding back. Don't let that skewed perception of yourself be something that keeps you from sharing how truly awesome you are with all of those in your personal circle of influence.

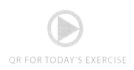

QR FOR TODAY'S EXERCISE

Do your thoughts about yourself prevent you from doing everything you can to be the best "you" possible? If so, how can you change your attitude?

THINK ABOUT THIS!

_____

_____

_____

_____

_____

PUT YOUR SITUATION IN PERSPECTIVE

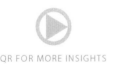

QR FOR MORE INSIGHTS

DESPITE WHAT I SAID ABOUT the news earlier, there's one good thing about it: i t sure makes you see that your situation probably isn't as bad as it could be, and when you become aware of how bad your life could be, it can be easier to see just how blessed you really are.

I mean, when was the last time a bomb came thundering through your house? Probably never! How often does a dictator control how you worship, what you can read, or who you can talk to? Most likely never! When was the last time you were in a plane crash? Probably never! And even if one or more of these situations apply to you, you have something to be grateful for—your existence, your family, the ability to build your life again. Some have it easier than others, but even in the direst circumstances, something could be worse.

Now, I know there are situations in your life that are tough. I have those, too; but when I think about how my life could be worse and put my issue into perspective on a case-by-case basis, I truly understand how blessed I am to live in this country and to have my health, a home, the love and support of my family, the opportunity to earn as much money as I want, the privilege to think as I choose, and the gift of my next breath. We really have to check ourselves when we start complaints like these:

- I hate my job.

- My kids drive me nuts.

- My wife is such a nag.

- It's too cold.

- It's too hot.

- Our house is ugly.

- I don't make enough money.

- My car is a piece of junk.

Seriously?!

Show gratitude for the things in your life that are going well and demonstrate a commitment (Remember Day 11?) to work on the things you'd like to change. Putting your life in perspective brings balance, just as putting all things in perspective will (as you'll see later). Often times, when our lives are out of perspective, we are out of balance; and we naturally tend to think on the negative side of

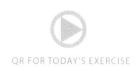

QR FOR TODAY'S EXERCISE

. . . when you become aware of how bad your life could be, it can be easier to see just how blessed you really are.

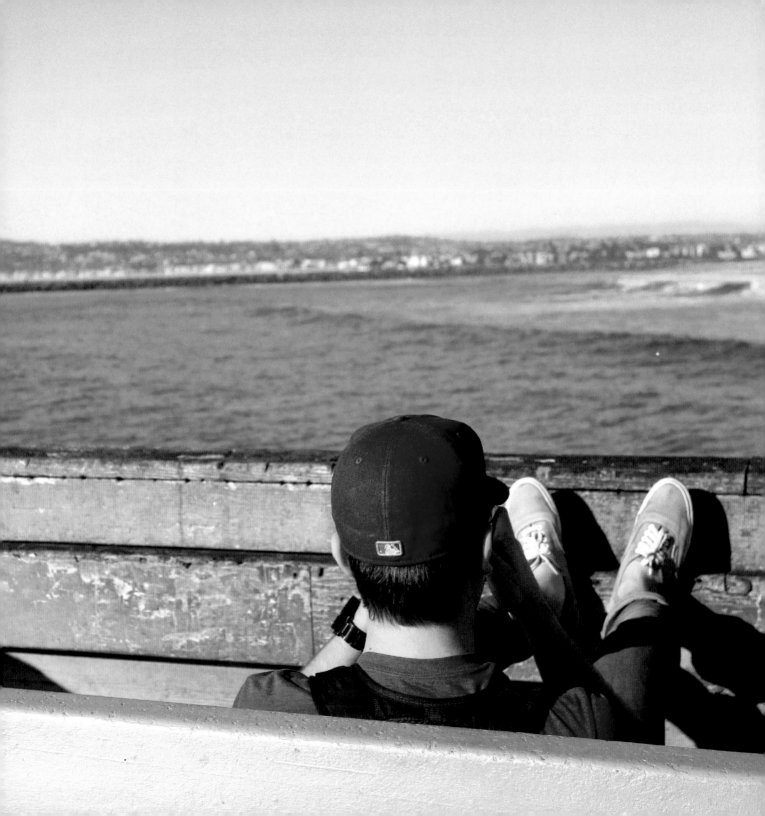

the equation as opposed to the positive. If we make adjustments to perspective continuously, it helps us see things differently, creating balance—a mental homeostasis where the body is at its healthiest.

So instead of whining and complaining, try saying things like, "I'm glad I'm working right now, and I hope I can get a better job soon." or "My wife and I aren't getting along so well. What can I do to improve our relationship?"

Only you can CHOOSE the things you say and think, so approach today by gaining perspective and being a little more appreciative of what you have. I have no clue what your life has consisted of to this point, but I encourage you to look at where you are RIGHT NOW, at this very second. Then ask yourself, "How are things in my life?" and find something you are grateful for.

Only you can CHOOSE the things you say and think...

Write down a list of everything in your life you like and then everything you complain about. Which is longer? How can you work to change your complaints or put them in perspective?

THINK ABOUT THIS!

_____

_____

_____

_____

_____

BE A HORSE, NOT A CAMEL

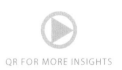

QR FOR MORE INSIGHTS

A **FEW YEARS BACK, I** spoke on an army base in Barstow, California. I had the honor of addressing a group of soldiers in an effort to motivate them to live drug- and alcohol-free and maintain a great attitude as they continued to serve this great country of ours.

Prior to speaking, I had a chance to tour the base. I took a walk through their museum, where I found the perfect analogy for my speech. Apparently, during the 1800s, the Army experimented with camels to see how they compared to horses. Here are some of the highlights:

Comparison: Horses vs. Camels

Could camels swim the Colorado River?

All 70 camels crossed without incident. Unfortunately, 8 horses and 14 mules drowned during the crossing.

How did the camels compare in cold weather?

In January, Lt. Beale pitched his camp within a few hundred yards of the summit of the Sierra Nevada Mountains. His camels thrived happily and grew fat in two to three feet of snow. During a snowstorm, camels were sent to rescue stranded wagons, people and mules. The camels brought the load through ice and snow back to camp. A strong, six-mule team was unable to extricate the empty wagons. Yet the camels seemed to pull them out with little effort. The camels were sent back to retrieve the mules, which were freezing to death. The mules were tied up on the sides of the camels and carried out of the snow and mountains.

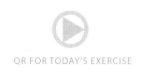

QR FOR TODAY'S EXERCISE

Would the camel's soft, leathery feet carry him across the stony [Southwestern] desert?

The camel has no shuffle in its gait, but lifts its foot perpendicularly from the ground and replaces it without sliding. The camel's coarsely granulated footpad enables it to travel continuously in a region where other beasts could not last a week.

How often do camels and horses need water?

A horse needs 8–12 gallons of water, 2–3 times a day in the desert. A camel can go 10–12 days without water. Horses need special foods, whereas camels eat almost any desert vegetation. Horses do not perform well under extreme heat or cold. Neither seems to affect camels.

How much of a load can a camel carry?

A horse can carry 170–250 pounds and walk 30–40 miles in a day with stops and watering. A camel was tested over several days with increasing load. The camel carried up to 1,256 pounds, 40–45 miles in a day at one continuous speed, but needed a day or two of rest. A 600–800 pound load was more acceptable for the camel and could be carried for several days.

How do camels compare for riding?

On a special trip away from camp, Lt. Beale rode his camel, Sid, eight miles an hour with "least effort" and traveled twenty-seven miles in three hours. Generally, a horse can travel 35 miles over an eight-hour period, but would need rest the next day.

Why did the camels fail the experiments?

In spite of the fact that they won most of the challenges, the camels scared the horses, mules and all the other animals in general. None of the soldiers could bond with a camel as well as they could bond with a horse. The camels bit, spat, and made noises.

Our attitude has a lot to do with our success and our growth...

Essentially, the Army decided not to use the camel because it had a bad attitude! And this happens with people, too. Our attitude has a lot to do with our success and our growth, and we're going to be exploring that more in the next couple of days. I've known countless people with amazing talents in business, sports and life in general who don't make it very far because they, too, have a rotten attitude.

THINK ABOUT THIS!

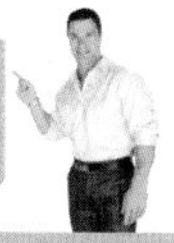

Has your attitude held you back from accomplishing things in life? If so, how will you make a change for the better?

_____

_____

_____

_____

_____

_____

_____

_____

_____

_____

_____

_____

_____

_____

DAY 24 CHANGE YOUR ATTITUDE, CHANGE YOUR LIFE

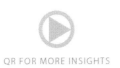

QR FOR MORE INSIGHTS

MY WHOLE CAREER AS A personal trainer, motivational speaker, author, model, TV host, and spokesperson has been devoted to helping people achieve the things they want most out of life. It's been a lot of fun, and the success stories of the people I've been able to help are incredibly rewarding, but I've noticed something that has really bugged me over the years: most people don't like to be corrected. Even when they seek correction from someone who knows what they're talking about, a bad attitude can put up a huge wall of resistance that's hard to overcome. With some people, nothing seems to work. And believe me, I try everything from a hardcore approach to being Mr. Nice Guy.

If you've gotten this far in my thirty-day program, you're probably not the type of person who puts up barriers to good advice. And that's great! I'm here to help you, and you're here to do what I tell you to do. It's nothing personal!

However, I want to make sure that this effective system is working for you in other areas of your life where a good attitude might be harder to come by. You've probably heard the saying "familiarity breeds contempt," for example. Simply put, it means that you get pissed off when your husband or wife says something like, "You shouldn't be eating those cookies if you're trying to lose weight."

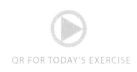

QR FOR TODAY'S EXERCISE

It's hard enough for people when I tell them that, and I'm not involved in their lives on a daily basis. So it's even more important to get a great attitude with the people you're closest to, like your spouse, boss, co-workers, kids, friends, pastor, religious leader, counselor, or parents. This will help you mellow out when they come to you with loving criticism that you know deep down you can benefit from. And it may even allow you to take their advice!

The process can be a painful one, but the rewards are really worth it. Your network of family, friends, colleagues, and coaches is there to help you be the best you can be, and if you close that network off, then you'll never change.

Do you accept easily constructive criticism from the people closest to you? Who sets you off the most and why? What can you do to change your attitude?

THINK ABOUT THIS!

_____

_____

_____

_____

25 # LEARN WHY PROBLEMS AREN'T YOUR PROBLEM

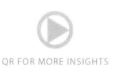

MORE OFTEN, IT'S YOUR ATTITUDE towards a perceived problem that's really your problem. Yes, I'm continuing the attitude theme because I think it's that big a deal! Actually, I could have invested the entire thirty days on this, but hopefully we can nail it in just a few.

A couple of days back we discussed perspective, and I'm going to revisit that a bit here also. Let's create a scenario to better help you understand perspective as it relates to your attitude toward any given situation.

I think this following note from a college student to her parents will help:

> *Dear Mom and Dad,*
>
> *Since I left for college, I know I've been remiss in writing. I'm sorry for my thoughtlessness, so I'm going to bring you up to date in this letter. Before you read it, please sit down. Are you sitting down? Please don't read this unless you're sitting down!*

Well, I'm getting along pretty well now. The skull fracture and concussion that I got when I jumped out the window when my dorm room caught on fire are pretty much healed. I only get those sick headaches once a day now.

Fortunately, an attendant at the gas station across the street witnessed the fire and the jump. He ran over to help me, took me to the hospital, and continued to visit me there. Once I got out of the hospital, I had nowhere to live because of the condition of my burnt-out room, so he invited me to share his basement apartment with him. It's sorta small, but really cute.

He's a very fine boy, and we've fallen deeply in love. We're planning to get married! We haven't set the exact date yet, but it will be before my pregnancy begins to show. Yes, Mom and Dad, I'm pregnant!

I know how much you're looking forward to being grandparents, and I know that you'll welcome the baby and give it the same tender care and devotion that you gave me when I was a child.

The reason for the delay in our marriage is that my boyfriend has a minor infection that I carelessly caught from him. I know you will welcome him into our family with open arms. After all, he's kind, and, although not well educated, ambitious. Although he's a different race and religion than we are, I know that your often-expressed tolerance will not permit you to be bothered by that.

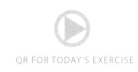

QR FOR TODAY'S EXERCISE

More often, it's your attitude towards a perceived problem that's really your problem.

Now that I've brought you up to date, I do want to tell you that there was no dorm fire, I don't have a concussion or skull fracture, I wasn't in the hospital, I'm not pregnant, I'm not infected, and there is no boyfriend in my life. However, I am failing history and science, and I wanted you to have a proper perspective!

How happy were those parents when they got to the end of that note? If their daughter had just said, "I'm failing history and science," they would have freaked out. But in relation to what they thought was happening to their child, failing a couple of subjects could easily be overcome.

Problems are as big as we make them, and we just give thoughts, fears, and negative emotions power by imagining and projecting things and by approaching them with a bad attitude. We must focus on being in the NOW and not living in the past. For example, I recently left a very high-paying job with no absolute replacement. Now, I could sit here and imagine what can go wrong all day, giving into negativity, or I can get to work on my future. I'm learning every day, as you should be, that it's all in how we see our problems and what action we take to overcome them that matters. It's all about our attitude and how we perceive our issues as either opportunities or walls.

I hope this letter made you smile and also made you realize how easy it is to make situations seem worse than they really are.

It's all about our attitude and how we perceive our issues as either opportunities or walls...

THINK ABOUT THIS!

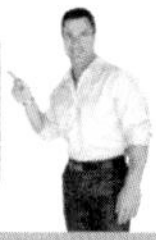

Do you overreact to "problems" and make mountains out of mole-hills? If so, what can you do to put your problems in their proper perspective?

_____

_____

_____

_____

_____

_____

_____

_____

_____

_____

_____

DAY 26

DON'T LET FALSE PRIDE KEEP YOU FROM REALLY BEING GREAT

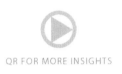

QR FOR MORE INSIGHTS

IF YOU CAN BALANCE PRIDE with perspective and gratitude, it can be one of the most endearing of all human qualities. Watching your son throw the winning touchdown or your daughter cross the finish line in first place and being humble in the sharing of that story for the next week is pride at its best. It's when we brag to the point of being obnoxious or demeaning—or worse—that we run into trouble and allow pride to get the best of us. Proverbs 16:18 says, "Pride goes before destruction, and a haughty spirit before a fall." Pride can hold you back from getting the things you want in life, even getting the body you've always dreamed of.

Pride is a double-edged sword that must be handled with the utmost caution and vigilance. It can be lethal and devastating to those who misuse it. It can hold you back from accepting constructive criticism and can cause others to resent you. Pride can cause you to think more highly of yourself than you should, and you could easily be passed over for a promotion as a result. Pride can take down heavyweight champions, world leaders, and superpowers.

They say that love is blind, but I think pride can leave you even more in the dark. Unhealthy pride is so obvious to the people around us, but we can't see it in ourselves most of the time. As you interact with others, check yourself during conversations. For one, don't dominate a conversation with what you've done, how good your kid is, what you know, or otherwise. It's beautiful when we say, "I heard little Johnny made the varsity baseball team. Can you tell me about that?" and do not interrupt with our story of little Sally and how she is the best dancer in class or how we were so good at baseball when we played it.

Also be aware of other situations where you might begin to think too highly of yourself. For example, the temptation to become prideful after becoming fit is there for many. I've seen relationships break apart because one spouse got fit, began to feel sexy again, and began to flaunt a new and improved version of themselves, feeling like they were better than their spouse.

Pride can affect every part of your life, so be aware of what you are doing and saying so you can become conscious of when you may be crossing into that unhealthy territory.

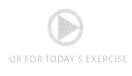

QR FOR TODAY'S EXERCISE

What are the things you're most proud of? What sense of perspective, humility, and gratitude can you bring to these things to ensure that your pride in them is balanced and healthy?

THINK ABOUT THIS!

_____

_____

_____

_____

DAY 27 — TAKE A DEEP BREATH

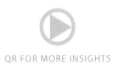

QR FOR MORE INSIGHTS

AS HARD AS WE TRY to be upbeat and positive, sometimes we get stressed, angry, and upset. None of us are impervious to these emotions, but that doesn't mean we can't learn to control them better so they don't rule us. There's a scripture in James 1:19 that says, "My dear brothers and sisters, take note of this: Everyone should be quick to listen, slow to speak, and slow to become angry." I can't tell you how many times I've repeated this in my head when I've been tempted to get mad, react negatively to a situation, or get engaged in an argument. It really can help you avoid conflict.

- Be quick to listen: this helps you from impulsively jumping to conclusions. If you listen before speaking, you'll have a better chance at understanding what the other person is trying to tell you.

- Be slow to speak: when confronted, it's important to avoid puking out the first thing that enters your mind. After you listen, take a moment to process the information so that you can say something you won't regret later.

- Be slow to become angry: if you listen first and then say something thoughtful, it's much easier not to get angry. You won't escalate the situation, and you'll often help calm the other person down. Or you may just see how unnecessary the situation is and find a way to exit gracefully.

You will ALWAYS end up in a better place if you refuse to let others engage you in a negative situation!

Another great tool you can use when you experience a negative emotion like fear or anger is deep breathing. A technique I use is to inhale as deeply as possible through my nose while starting to say something in my head like a scripture or positive statement and to exhale while finishing the statement. For example, you might say to yourself, "For God did not give me a spirit of fear" . . . on the inhale and then ". . . but one of love, power, and a sound mind." on the exhale. Another one I use is "I am strong, confident, and fearful of nothing." Do this with the statement of your choice and watch how easy it is to rise above any uncomfortable situation. Just make

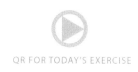

QR FOR TODAY'S EXERCISE

You will ALWAYS end up in a better place if you refuse to let others "engage" you in a negative situation!

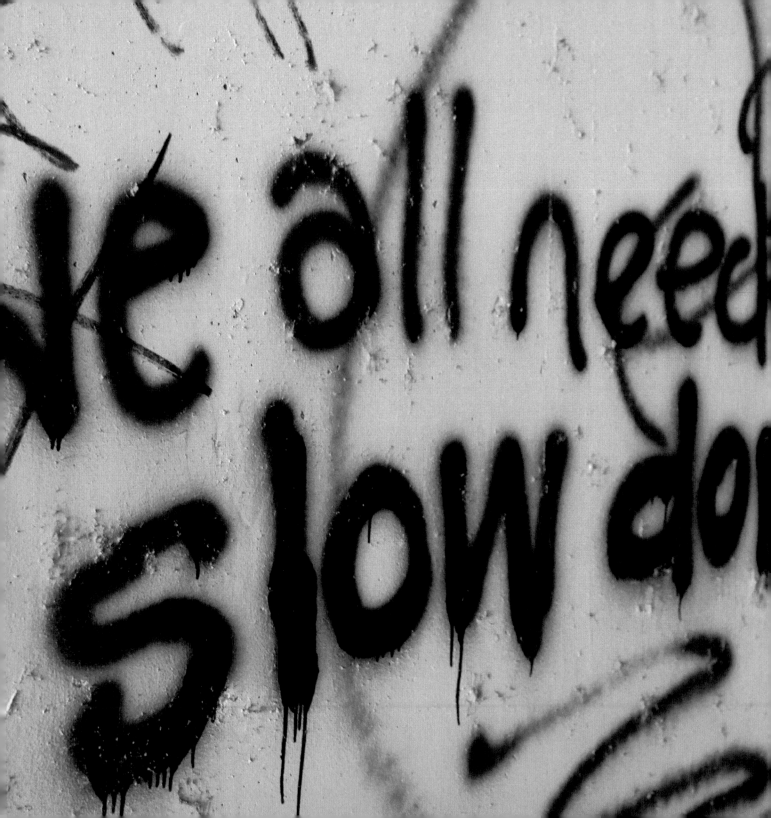

it a bold statement of positivity that will help you overcome whatever situation you are facing.

The more you begin to eliminate negative emotions and actions in your life, the more you'll give yourself the freedom to experience life to the fullest.

THINK ABOUT THIS!

Write down all the situations where a deep breath came in handy today.

_____

_____

_____

_____

_____

_____

_____

_____

_____

_____

_____

DAY 28

SHARE YOUR EXPERTISE

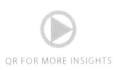

QR FOR MORE INSIGHTS

ABOUT TEN YEARS AGO, a close friend of mine challenged me to commit to my personal growth. I didn't really get it at first, to be honest. I thought to myself, "I'm pretty motivated, and I'm not stupid, so why do I need personal growth?" Well, once I started, I quickly realized how important continuous improvement is to me as a husband, father, and businessman.

Part of the challenge my friend gave me was to get up and speak to different groups of people. This was tough, and sometimes I still get nervous when I think about speaking in public, but I never allow that to stop me. I just face it and get out there in faith, and it's amazing every time. One of the best things about speaking is being able to change people's lives—from high school students to prison inmates—and if I gave into that fear, I'd never be able to reach anybody on such a personal level. Sharing my expertise has been

96

incredibly rewarding, has changed my life for the better, and opened up my spirit in countless ways.

I want you to take the challenge to speak to and inspire others. Share your talents and the things you're passionate about with people, and it will help you as much as it helps them. Just talk about the things you know. It could be about your job, your hobbies, parenting skills, funny stories about your dog, anything that could be of interest to kids, parents, professionals, or members of local organizations like the Rotary Club. If you live in a city, see if there's an "Ignite" group available. They give you strict parameters for giving your presentation, which might make it easier. Or look into organizations like Toastmasters, where you can practice your skills with a friendly audience.

Just getting yourself out there and offering your knowledge to others will take you places you never imagined. It will stretch you to the point that you have to grow, and you'll be better off as a result.

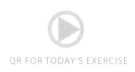

QR FOR TODAY'S EXERCISE

Is something inside you that you should share with others and haven't because of fear? Write down some possible topics and commit to discussing them in front of a group within the next month.

THINK ABOUT THIS!

_____

_____

_____

_____

_____

DAY 29 ACT LIKE IT'S YOUR LAST DAY ON EARTH

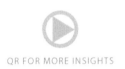

QR FOR MORE INSIGHTS

I'M NOT TRYING TO BE MORBID here, but what if today was your last day on Earth? Would you have said what you said to your spouse? Child? Co-Worker? Yourself? Would you have gone to bed angry last night or wasted one minute complaining about useless things that actually mean nothing?

How many days have you wasted over the last year gossiping about, envying or possibly even hating something or someone? If you sit back and really think on this for a minute, you'll easily see that you've wasted precious time and energy on things that you wouldn't even give a second thought about if this were your last day on the planet.

Think about how quickly you blazed through school and moved on to live your own life. How fast have the years passed? How fast have you hit your twenty-first birthday or your thirtieth or fiftieth? These milestones come and go so quickly, but what was your quality of life at each of these stages? Did you enjoy that time or waste it by having a poor, unappreciative attitude? How much regret do you have?

Try this: each day for the next week, act as if it's your last. Say things to people that you always wished you had. Enjoy quality time with the people who mean the most to you. Invest in someone else's life by imparting some wisdom that was passed on to you. Just LIVE for the next seven days.

Of course, do it all in a positive way: don't go rob a bank or cuss out your boss because it's probably not your last day on Earth, and that's obviously a giant step in the wrong direction! But you get the point. We only have so many days to fully live out our lives, so why would we want to live them any other way than joyfully and with gratitude and thankfulness for all that we've been given? When you put it all in perspective, all of this becomes so much easier.

My hope is that you enjoy many more days on this Earth, and I also hope that those days are ones that you enjoy and live to the fullest.

QR FOR TODAY'S EXERCISE

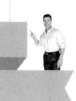

THINK ABOUT THIS!

As you live each day as if it were your last, write down some of the reactions you get from people. How does living this way change your life?

_____

_____

_____

_____

DAY 30
ENJOY THE JOURNEY AS MUCH AS THE DESTINATION

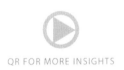

QR FOR MORE INSIGHTS

I'VE MENTIONED FOCUSING MORE ON the process than the outcome before, and I want to delve into that idea a little deeper today. We're often taught when it comes to a goal to focus only on the objective, to just go for it without paying attention to what's around us. This is exactly the opposite of what I feel we should be doing. It's important not to get distracted, but we also have to be open to everything around us.

Another way of saying it is to "stop and smell the roses." The thing is that your journey won't, and shouldn't, happen overnight. Don't put stress on yourself—as stress kills and slows progress on weight loss and fitness goals. If we learn to relax through this ENTIRE process, it makes the ride way more enjoyable, and it becomes all about the beauty in the process and the journey. Don't miss out on all the beautiful things that surround you on your way to where you want to be!

As you work towards the realization of your goals, understand that each and every moment of that process holds something within it that you can use for your development and satisfaction or as a life lesson that will benefit someone else in your circle of influence. You must simply DECIDE to look for the blessing in each situation, person, and experience you encounter along the way. There goes that "decide" word again. It really is that easy!

I'm not going to beat this one up. Instead, I'm going to let you start enjoying the process of growth by putting all you've learned into practice today.

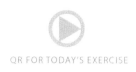

QR FOR TODAY'S EXERCISE

THINK ABOUT THIS!

Expand your awareness and write down some of the pleasant surprises you encounter today.

_____

_____

_____

_____

_____

_____

NEXT STEPS

CELEBRATE HOW FAR YOU'VE COME—AND KEEP GOING FURTHER!

CONGRATULATIONS! YOU'VE FINISHED this thirty-day journey toward success, and I'm excited to have walked alongside you the entire time.

Over the last thirty days, you've been evolving in many exciting ways, reprogramming your mind for optimal performance, perfectly practicing things that make you better, and so many other things. It's virtually impossible to have come this far without making significant progress.

I know I'm a totally different man than I was thirty days ago. Writing this book has made me more open to correction, more appreciative of all that I have, more willing to overcome fear and anxiety, and more prepared to give without expectation. Even if you're not exactly where you want to be, you can be thankful that you're not where you used to be. And if you continue along the path, you'll make even greater progress.

Without getting too philosophical, I'll leave you with what I feel is my best advice as we part ways. In the immortal words of Sir Winston Churchill, "Never, never, never, never give up!"

Even if you're not exactly where you want to be, you can be thankful that you're not where you used to be

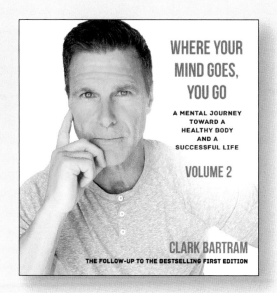

INSPIRED BY HIS READERS' REQUESTS for additional information on the topics contained in this revised edition, Clark has compiled another thirty days of steps to guide you on your mental journey in a new companion book titled *Where Your Mind Goes, You Go, Volume 2*. Order it today to continue moving your life in a positive direction.

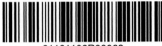
Made in the USA
Middletown, DE
17 August 2019